THE QUICK AND EASY
IBS RELIEF COOKBOOK

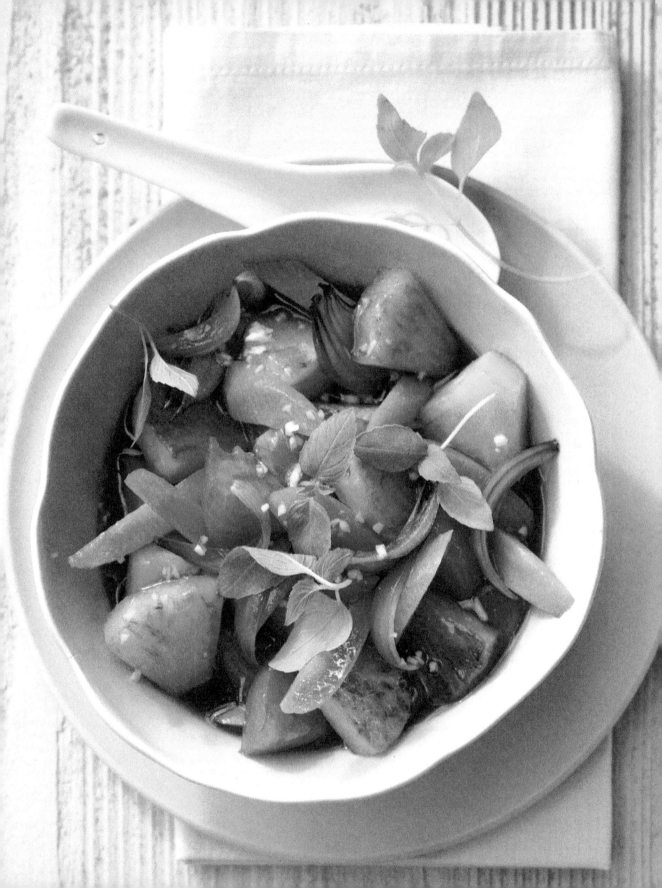

THE QUICK *and* EASY
IBS Relief
COOKBOOK

Over 120 Low-FODMAP Recipes to
Soothe Irritable Bowel Syndrome Symptoms

KAREN FRAZIER

ROCKRIDGE
PRESS

For general information on our other products and services or to obtain technical support, please contact our Customer Care Department within the United States at (866) 744-2665, or outside the United States at (510) 253-0500.

Rockridge Press publishes its books in a variety of electronic and print formats. Some content that appears in print may not be available in electronic books, and vice versa.

TRADEMARKS: Rockridge Press and the Rockridge Press logo are trademarks or registered trademarks of Callisto Media Inc., and/or its affiliates, in the United States and other countries, and may not be used without written permission. All other trademarks are the property of their respective owners. Rockridge Press is not associated with any product or vendor mentioned in this book.

Front cover photography © Tara Donne/Offset; donatas1205/Shutterstock

Back cover photography © Jan-Peter Westermann/ Stockfood; Great Stock!/Stockfood; Martí Sans/Stocksy

Interior photography © Jan-Peter Westermann/Stockfood, p.ii; James Jackson/Stocksy, p.vi; Helen Rushbrook/Stocksy, p.xii; Gräfe & Unzer Verlag/Kramp + Gölling/Stockfood, p.24; Gillian Vann/Stocksy, p.42; Gräfe & Unzer Verlag/ Kramp + Gölling/Stockfood, p.58; Eising Studio - Food Photo & Video/Stockfood, p.74; Gräfe & Unzer Verlag/Jörn Rynio/ Stockfood, p.92; Great Stock!/Stockfood, p.110; Martí Sans/ Stocksy, p.132; Gräfe & Unzer Verlag/Kramp + Gölling/ Stockfood, p.148; The Picture Pantry/Stockfood, p.168

ISBN: Print 978-1-62315-924-5| eBook 978-1-62315-925-2

For my mom, Brenda,
whose recipes I've blatantly copied
from time to time over the years.

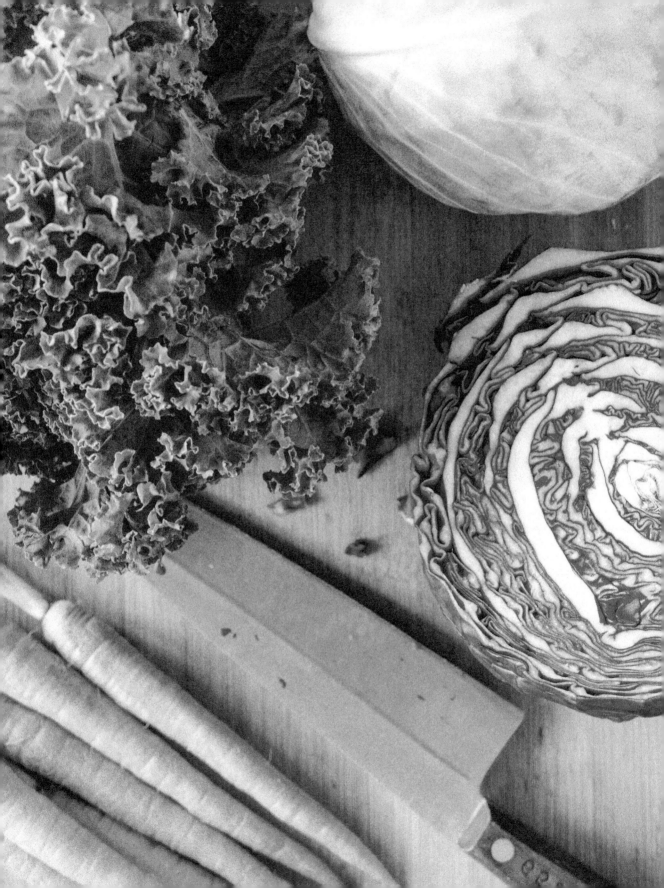

CONTENTS

FOREWORD

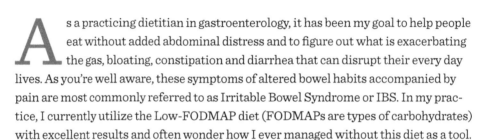

A s a practicing dietitian in gastroenterology, it has been my goal to help people eat without added abdominal distress and to figure out what is exacerbating the gas, bloating, constipation and diarrhea that can disrupt their every day lives. As you're well aware, these symptoms of altered bowel habits accompanied by pain are most commonly referred to as Irritable Bowel Syndrome or IBS. In my practice, I currently utilize the Low-FODMAP diet (FODMAPs are types of carbohydrates) with excellent results and often wonder how I ever managed without this diet as a tool.

The rate of IBS diagnosis is on the rise as more and more people are headed to the doctor to seek help. But we need to look at *how* we eat as well as the foods we choose when trying to figure out the culprits of our altered digestion. The amount of wheat (fructans) we ingest has tripled over the years and the type of highly refined flours is predominantly present in our breads, pasta, cookies and cakes. These items are also commonly sweetened with a readily available and inexpensive sweetener: high fructose corn syrup (HFCS) and can act as double trouble on the gut (fructose). In order to keep up with the demand for processed foods in our increasingly busy lifestyles, the packaged foods being developed are adding to our tummy troubles as the FODMAP content soars. We also are finding that our hectic schedules allow for less time to calmly sit down to a home-cooked meal.

Food, although not the cause of IBS, can increase IBS-related symptoms and it has been challenging to uncover intolerances until the Low-FODMAP diet was developed around 2005. For some people, the consumption of high-FODMAP foods will increase bloating and cause visceral hypersensitivity. It was a painstaking process of trial and error until the research of Sue Shepherd, Peter Gibson, and the team at Monash University developed a scientifically based strategy of elimination and reintroduction of foods to help people identify those triggers and coined the term the Low-FODMAP Diet. When these problematic foods are removed, symptoms essentially disappear and life no longer involves a battle to get out of the house or frantically trying to find the nearest restroom. The Low-FODMAP diet is now a well-known method for managing gastrointestinal distress, by changing what we eat. Also, it empowers us to manage our relationship with food in the most natural way.

In order to implement the Low-FODMAP diet, you need guidance and the right tools. Having a good resource and cookbook to guide you along the process of elimination and reintroduction is critical. In this book, Karen Frazier walks you through the different phases of the diet in a user-friendly way, to help to uncover all the triggers that can upset your GI tract and interfere with your daily life. Within, you'll find tips and tricks for organizing yourself to start and stick to a Low-FODMAP diet, and easy, delicious recipes using the freshest, minimally processed ingredients, to keep your gut happy. Karen's approach will help you find you way back to the joy of cooking and eating.

LAURA MANNING, MPH, RDN, CDN
Clinical Nutrition Coordinator
Susan and Leonard Feinstein
Inflammatory Bowel Disease Center
Mount Sinai Medical Center

INTRODUCTION

It can feel incredibly frustrating to suffer from gastrointestinal distress brought about by irritable bowel syndrome (IBS) pain. I understand. While I don't have IBS, I was diagnosed with it at one point based on my symptoms alone. It turned out, though, I have celiac disease (something that took almost 25 years to diagnose properly), so I can relate to the severity of pain and the discomfort. There were days I didn't leave my house (and barely left the bathroom) because of the gastrointestinal issues I experienced.

Once you receive an accurate diagnosis, especially if you've been pursuing one for a while, there's an immediate feeling of relief. You think: *Whew—finally, I know what I'm dealing with! I'm not crazy. It has a name, and it's a real thing.* Often, however, that feeling of relief is followed quickly by a new thought.

What do I do now?

Your health-care provider most likely told you one of the best ways to manage your symptoms was with a low-FODMAP diet. And, suddenly, your excitement at having a proper diagnosis deflates as you realize you are going from one set of restrictions to another—having to monitor every bite of food you take to keep symptoms at bay.

The thought of adopting a restrictive diet for your health can be daunting as you begin to realize that gone are the days of casual dining, grabbing something quickly on the go, or eating the premade foods that make life more convenient.

When I first switched to my new self-defense diet (which is what I called it back in the day), I was frustrated. I felt like I'd gone from spending all my time in the bathroom to spending all my time shopping for and preparing food. Now, I like cooking, but I also had a busy life including a full-time career and young children with a zillion activities, so the thought of spending hours shopping and cooking every day stressed me out (not a good thing for my symptoms, either). Not only that, but for a while it kept me from pursuing a nutritional solution to my celiac disease. Instead of eating the way I should, I kept convenience at the fore and suffered ongoing and nearly debilitating symptoms.

If you recognize yourself in my story, I have good news. You *can* have both. You can manage your symptoms through your diet and free up your time—with less stress—by preparing quick and easy low-FODMAP recipes that are as tasty as they are simple.

And that is exactly what the recipes in this cookbook are designed to do: free you from spending hours at the grocery store and in the kitchen. Instead, these recipes are designed with simplicity in mind. Each recipe has either five or fewer main ingredients, or takes no more than 30 minutes to prepare from start to finish. For those that do take a little longer to prepare, most of the time is inactive so you can do other things as the food cooks or chills.

IBS has many triggers, and stress is one. For many, having to shop for and prepare a specialized diet adds to that stress. With these easy recipes at your fingertips, you can nourish yourself with flavorful foods that support your gastrointestinal health—and without all that time spent shopping and cooking you are free to pursue the activities you enjoy. These recipes will not only will result in more free time while helping you manage your symptoms with diet, but they will also help relieve some stress. You will have time to savor delicious foods and life's pleasures and joys—essential elements to healing your body and spirit.

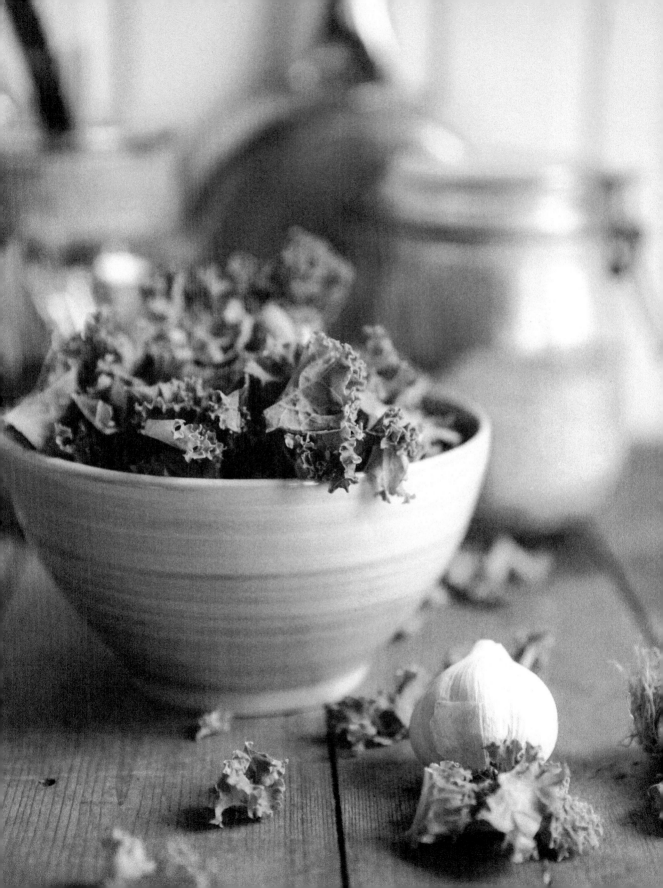

ONE

Managing Irritable Bowel Syndrome through Diet

Here you are. You now know which diet to follow that will bring relief from your IBS symptoms. But how effective is it? It depends on whom you ask and which studies you read. A recent study in *The Journal of Clinical and Experimental Gastroenterology* suggests that, on average, 9 out of 10 patients diagnosed with IBS who follow a low-FODMAP diet experience improvement in overall symptoms. To understand how it helps, it's necessary to look at the mechanics of IBS and how ingesting foods containing FODMAPs affects your symptoms.

What Is IBS?

According to the International Foundation for Functional Gastrointestinal Disorders (IFFGD), irritable bowel syndrome, or IBS, is a functional gastrointestinal disorder. In this disorder, the gastrointestinal system doesn't function as it should. It is characterized by a range of gastrointestinal symptoms, such as diarrhea, constipation, alternating diarrhea and constipation, abdominal cramping and pain, and gas and bloating. In some cases of IBS, bouts of these symptoms appear frequently and may be quite debilitating. It's likely you're painfully familiar with most or all of these.

IBS is a *syndrome*. Dictionary.com defines a syndrome as a group of symptoms that occur together and characterize a specific disease or condition. In many cases, doctors and medical professionals lack a full understanding of the underlying causes. In fact, a syndrome may be a complex collection of symptoms stemming from multiple causes—which means both the cause and reactions may be different depending on the person.

Diagnosis of a syndrome usually occurs after excluding other causes of symptoms with testing, which means it can take quite a while to arrive at that diagnosis. With this in mind, there are three main types of IBS characterized by symptoms:

1. **IBS-C:** constipation dominant

2. **IBS-D:** diarrhea dominant

3. **IBS alternating type:** characterized by alternating bouts of constipation and diarrhea

CAUSES AND TRIGGERS

According to the Mayo Clinic, the cause of IBS is poorly understood, although theories exist as to its underlying factors.

COMMUNICATION WITH THE BRAIN AND INTESTINAL TRACT

One of the main theories regarding the cause of IBS is faulty communication between the brain and the intestinal tract. This abnormal communication may result in intestinal spasms, which then speed or slow the movement of stools through the intestines while causing cramping and discomfort.

INTESTINAL SENSITIVITY

Another underlying cause of IBS may be overly sensitive intestines that are more likely to react to certain factors, including:

- Hormones
- Illness
- Medications
- Stress
- Various foods

BACTERIAL OR YEAST OVERGROWTH

As noted by the Digestive Health Institute, another theory suggests IBS may be caused by an autoimmune disease. In this case, some studies suggest a previous gastrointestinal infection triggers small intestinal bacterial overgrowth (SIBO), which stimulates antibodies in the intestines and causes the immune system to attack the intestines.

Functional medicine specialist Dr. Amy Myers also notes yeast overgrowth can cause symptoms similar to IBS, which may point to another potential cause.

FACTORS THAT WORSEN IBS

Many people discover there are certain things that cause their IBS symptoms to worsen. Therefore, controlling these factors may help minimize or eliminate symptoms and flare-ups of the syndrome.

FODMAPS

Researchers at Australia's Monash University discovered that ingesting foods containing FODMAPS caused an increase in IBS symptoms, and reducing or eliminating these foods brought relief from symptoms in a significant percentage of their patients. FODMAPs appear in numerous fruits, vegetables, grains, and other foods (see pages 5 and 6 for more information). Avoiding these foods brings significant reduction in symptoms in about 86 percent of patients with IBS.

FOOD ALLERGY

According to Food Allergy Research and Education (FARE), a food allergy is an immune system response to proteins in certain foods. When you eat the foods, the body misinterprets their presence as a foreign pathogen and responds by creating antibodies to fight them off. About 3.5 to 4 percent of the US population has some type of food allergy. Food allergies, unlike food intolerances (see next page) can result in life-threatening symptoms. *Avoid any foods you know you are allergic to.*

An October 2004 article in the medical journal *Gut* examined the relationship between food allergy and IBS, noting IBS symptoms have factors in common with food allergies, such as how impairment to the gut's barrier interacts with unusual immune function. The article also notes a relationship between allergic antibodies and IBS symptoms. This indicates there may be a relationship between the two. The eight most common food allergens include:

1. Cow's milk and other dairy products
2. Eggs
3. Fish
4. Peanuts
5. Shellfish
6. Soy
7. Tree nuts
8. Wheat

FOOD INTOLERANCE

The IBS Network notes people with IBS often have intolerances to foods that cause symptoms. More common than food allergies, food intolerances are *not* an immune system response as allergies are, but rather are functional and symptomatic responses caused by the body's inability to process certain foods. According to Allergy UK, these intolerances may be caused by a number of factors, including certain medications, histamines in certain foods, enzyme defects, and food additives or toxins.

FOOD SENSITIVITY

Sensitivities to different foods may also affect IBS symptoms. Sensitivities are milder forms of intolerances, so reactions may be less severe than with intolerances or allergies, but in cases of symptomatic IBS, avoiding foods to which you are sensitive may help reduce symptoms.

CELIAC DISEASE

Celiac disease is an autoimmune condition in which the body reacts poorly to the consumption of gluten (found in wheat, barley, and rye, along with the many foods that contain these). With celiac disease, consumption of even trace amounts of gluten—some people are sensitive up to 25 ppm (parts per million) or more—causes the immune system to attack the intestinal villi, the small fingerlike projections that allow for nutrient absorption. The Celiac Disease Foundation notes celiac disease symptoms are very similar to IBS symptoms and, in cases where the conditions occur together, you will not be able to get your IBS symptoms under control until you've completely eliminated gluten from your diet. However, some people

Understanding FODMAPs

FODMAPs are a type of carbohydrate that may be difficult for the body to absorb. Because of this difficulty with absorption, consuming foods containing FODMAPs may trigger the gastrointestinal distress associated with IBS.

FODMAP is an acronym that stands for the different types of difficult-to-absorb carbohydrates.

FERMENTABLE These carbohydrates combine with bacteria in the lower intestinal tract and ferment there. According to Hamilton Health Sciences, fermentable carbs include those that contain lactose (a milk sugar), and are found in:

- Many dairy products, such as cow's milk and cream

- Fructans (foods that contain fructose chains), which are found in wheat

- Galactans (which contain chains of a sugar called galactose) such as legumes, onions, and peas

- Polyols, or sugar alcohols, found in apples, mushrooms, pears, and sweet corn

OLIGOSACCHARIDES These carbohydrates are made up of simple sugar chains and include fructans and galactans. Some foods in this category include artichokes, cereals made from wheat or rye, legumes, and watermelon.

DISACCHARIDES Foods containing a double sugar molecule, such as lactose found in dairy products.

MONOSACCHARIDES Some foods containing a single sugar molecule. For example, foods that contain excess fructose, which is a mono-saccharide, may be difficult to digest. Some foods with excess fructose include corn syrup, garlic, honey, maple syrup, onions, and peanuts.

AND That's all the A stands for—just a way to make it an easy-to-say acronym.

POLYOLS Foods that contain sugar alcohols, such as xylitol, mannitol, and erythritol.

→

CATEGORIES OF FODMAPS

Although the preceding categories make a pretty slick acronym, it's easier to classify FODMAPs by the *types* of sugars they contain.

The granddaddy of FODMAP research, Monash University, has a fantastic smartphone app—the Monash University Low-FODMAP Diet app—that helps you identify high- and low-FODMAP foods with a searchable database. It breaks down FODMAPs as follows:

OLIGOSACCHARIDES (OLIGOS)
Fructans and galactans
(see preceding)

FRUCTOSE Most fruits and vegetables contain fructose. The key is to find those that do *not* contain excessive amounts to help keep your FODMAP load low.

POLYOLS Sugar alcohols (see preceding). Note that many diabetic candies and sugarless gums contain polyols, as do certain low-carb sweeteners, like Truvia and Swerve.

LACTOSE Milk sugars, found in highest concentrations in cow's milk and some cheeses.

HOW FODMAPS EXACERBATE IBS

According to *Gastroenterology and Hepatology*, FODMAPs may exacerbate IBS symptoms because they are particularly difficult for the body to absorb. This causes fermentation in the intestines, as well as an increase in water to the bowels, which may result in gas, bloating, pain, reduced movement, spasms, and diarrhea or constipation.

Not all FODMAPs irritate everyone with IBS, so the best approach is total elimination for 30 days, followed by reintroduction of one category at a time to determine your personal triggers. Likewise, since it is impossible to entirely eliminate FODMAPs (unless you eat an entirely carb-free diet), what is important to focus on is FODMAP load, or the amount of FODMAPs you take in over the course of a meal, day, or week. Therefore, to keep your FODMAP load low, you need to eliminate foods particularly high in FODMAPs and, instead, choose lower-FODMAP foods.

with celiac disease continue to suffer from symptoms even after eliminating gluten completely from their diet. In these cases, the two conditions may coexist, requiring elimination of *both* gluten and FODMAPs to help control symptoms completely.

ACID REFLUX

According to Everyday Health, as many as three out of four people with IBS may also experience gastroesophageal reflux disease (GERD), or vice versa. Both are digestive tract disorders. A 2009 study from *Digestive Diseases and Sciences* concludes, "A first diagnosis of either IBS or GERD significantly increases the risk of a subsequent diagnosis of the other condition," suggesting one may be a factor in developing the other.

STRESS

IFFGD notes there is an increased gastrointestinal response to stress. Because stress stimulates the intestinal tract, it may lead to IBS symptoms. When the intestinal tract is stimulated, it affects movement and sensation in the intestines as well. So, all types of stress may worsen IBS symptoms.

KEEPING THE FACTORS IN CHECK

The recipes in this book are all designed to keep the worsening factors in check to help minimize or reduce IBS symptoms. The recipes, both simple and delicious:

- are all low in FODMAPs
- offer tips to help you avoid foods to which you are allergic, intolerant, or sensitive
- contain suggestions for variations to decrease acid reflux and gastroesophageal reflux disease
- are quick and easy, using easy-to-find ingredients—often only five or fewer—or taking fewer than 30 minutes total (or, in some cases, both) to reduce stress from time spent shopping for and preparing meals
- are gluten-free for people with celiac disease

The Question of Stress

If you've ever noticed your symptoms increase when you're under stress, you're not alone. Stress can have a profound effect on IBS symptoms, according to Melissa G. Hunt, PhD, author of *Reclaim Your Life from IBS*. In her book, Dr. Hunt suggests a technique called cognitive behavior therapy (CBT) to help relieve stress arising from negative thoughts, feelings, and moods that may contribute to your overall stress.

If you frequently don't feel well, it's natural to have negative thoughts, feelings, and moods associated with how IBS affects your life. Unfortunately, these feelings create further stress, which can further exacerbate symptoms, leading to a spiral of stress and symptoms. CBT seeks to help you break out of this cycle.

CBT is typically pursued within a therapeutic environment as a short-term way to break the cycle of habitual stressful or negative thoughts and feelings. However, although CBT is best pursued within a professional therapeutic setting, you can practice the following techniques to help you relieve and manage your everyday stress:

1. Monitor your thoughts.
2. Record negative events and your reactions to them.
3. Practice self-compassion.
4. Challenge and restructure negative thoughts.
5. Practice mindfulness meditation.

MONITOR YOUR THOUGHTS

The first step to eliminating habitual negative thoughts is to notice them. Pay attention to what you think, feel, and say. How often do you catch yourself thinking even minor negative thoughts? Start simply, by just noticing the thoughts that flit through your head. That's it. Just notice.

RECORD NEGATIVE EVENTS AND YOUR REACTIONS TO THEM

Divide a piece of paper into three columns. For three minutes at the end of each day, write a list in the first column of stressful or negative situations that occurred. In the second column, write a few single-word descriptions of how you feel about that event, such as "stressed," or "worried." In the third column, rate each descriptor on a scale of 0 (none) to 100 (extreme). Put the list away for 24 hours.

After a day, look at the list again and evaluate how extreme or distorted your thoughts may have been in relation to the actual situation. Look for patterns in your thinking, such as catastrophic thinking or experiencing overly negative reactions.

PRACTICE SELF-COMPASSION

It's easy to be compassionate to others, and much more difficult to show our-selves the same love and understanding. As you monitor your thoughts, practice self-compassion. Whenever you notice a pattern of negative or difficult thinking, or if you make a mistake, take a moment to treat yourself compassionately. So, if you make a mistake, rather than thinking something like, "I'm so stupid," talk to yourself supportively, as you would another person you care for. Ask yourself: What would you tell someone you love if they made a mistake? Then, have that conversation—with yourself.

CHALLENGE AND RESTRUCTURE NEGATIVE THOUGHTS

I'm a huge fan of The Work by Byron Katie (see Resources, page 170). In The Work, you take negative or judgmental thoughts and subject them to a process called *inquiry*. For each thought, you ask yourself a series of questions:

- Is it true? Can you possibly know, 100 percent, that it's true?

- How do you react when you believe that thought?

- Who would you be without that thought? What would your life look like without that thought?

    The next step is to turn the thought around to see if you can find another statement that would be just as true, or truer, than your original statement.

    For example, if your original thought was "I always mess up."

- **Is it true?** No—you don't always mess up 100 percent of the time.

- **How do you react when you believe it?** Probably not very well. It makes you angry at yourself or stressed.

- **Who would you be without the thought?** You'd probably be less stressed or frustrated.

- **Turn it around in a way that is as true, or truer, than your original statement.** Possible turnarounds are "I don't always mess up," or "I always do my best and it often comes out okay." Are both of these statements as true, or truer, than your original statement?

PRACTICE MINDFULNESS MEDITATION

By staying focused in the present moment and paying attention to your thoughts and feelings without judgment, you can break the pattern of harmful or destructive thoughts. Mindfulness meditation is simple, and you can do it for just five minutes a few times a day. To engage in mindfulness meditation:

1. Sit quietly and focus on your breathing.

2. Watch your thoughts as they arise. When they do, welcome them, then let them go without getting caught up in any emotion or judgment. No matter what arises, watch it without judgment and let it float away.

You can also practice mindfulness in everyday activities. For example, if you are doing dishes, pay attention to what you are doing. Notice the warm water on your hands, the sounds of the dishes, the scent of the dish soap. If you notice outside thoughts intruding, allow them to drift away and refocus your attention on the activity you are pursuing in the moment.

THE RECIPE FOR STRESS RELIEF

Cooking—especially when following a restrictive diet—can feel stressful, which is one of the reasons for this book. These recipes are designed to be simple and pleasurable. As you prepare them, focus on the foods and the process—the rhythm of chopping, the aromas of fresh herbs, the sizzle of a pan. Practice mindfulness while making these simple and flavorful recipes to help reduce stress even further.

FODMAP Food Charts

Since you don't want to guess which foods contain high levels of FODMAPs, which ones might be okay to have in small amounts, and which ones you can eat freely, the following charts can help you discern the best ways to eat as you follow a FODMAP elimination diet. You can also find this information in the handy smartphone app: The Monash University Low-FODMAP Diet.

High-FODMAP Foods to Avoid

DAIRY

- Buttermilk
- Cream cheese
- Custard
- Halloumi (cheese)
- Ice cream
- Milk: cow's, goat's, soy
- Pudding
- Sour cream
- Yogurt

FRUIT

- Apple
- Apricot
- Blackberries
- Boysenberries
- Cherries
- Figs
- Grapefruit
- Guava (unripened)
- Lychee
- Mango
- Nectarine
- Peach
- Pear
- Persimmon
- Plum
- Pomegranate
- Watermelon

VEGETABLES

- Artichokes: globe, Jerusalem
- Asparagus
- Beet
- Cabbage, savoy
- Cassava
- Cauliflower
- Corn, sweet
- Garlic
- Leek (white part only)
- Mushrooms
- Onion
- Peas
- Shallots
- Sweet potato
- Taro root
- Yucca

GRAINS/CEREALS

- Amaranth
- Barley
- Bread: multi-grain, rye, wheat
- Couscous
- Einkorn
- Emmer
- Granola
- Muesli
- Pasta, wheat
- Rice Krispies
- Rye
- Spelt
- Wheat
- Wheat bran

LEGUMES

- Beans of all kinds except chickpeas and lentils

NUTS/SEEDS

- Cashews
- Pistachios

HERBS/SPICES

- Chicory root (inulin)
- Garlic powder
- Onion powder

SWEETENERS

- Agave
- Honey
- Sugar alcohols

CONDIMENTS

- Ketchup
- Relish
- Tzatziki

Low-FODMAP Foods to Enjoy

DAIRY

**2 to 3 servings per day;
1 serving = ½ cup**

- Cheese: Brie, Camembert, Cheddar, feta, mozzarella, Parmesan, Swiss
- Ice cream (lactose-free)
- Milk: almond, coconut (canned), lactose-free, rice
- Yogurt: goat's milk, Greek-style, lactose-free

FRUIT

**2 to 3 servings per day;
1 serving = 1 medium
piece or 1 cup diced**

- Banana, ½
- Blueberries
- Breadfruit
- Cantaloupe
- Clementine
- Dragon fruit
- Durian
- Grapes
- Guava (ripe)
- Honeydew melon
- Kiwi
- Kumquat
- Lemon
- Lime
- Mandarin orange
- Orange
- Passion fruit
- Pawpaw
- Pineapple
- Plantain
- Prickly pear
- Raspberries
- Rhubarb
- Star fruit
- Strawberries
- Tamarind

VEGETABLES

**5 to 7 servings per day;
1 serving = 1 cup raw or
½ cup cooked**

- Arugula
- Beans, green
- Bean sprouts
- Bell pepper: green, red
- Bok choy
- Broccoli
- Brussels sprouts
- Cabbage: green, red
- Carrot
- Celery root (celeriac)
- Chicory leaves
- Chile pepper: green, red
- Collard greens
- Cucumber
- Eggplant
- Endive
- Fennel
- Kale
- Leek (green parts only)
- Lettuce
- Okra
- Olives
- Parsnip
- Pickles
- Potato, white
- Radicchio
- Radish
- Scallion (green parts only)
- Seaweed
- Spinach
- Squash: spaghetti, summer, zucchini
- Swiss chard
- Tomato
- Turnip

GRAINS/CEREALS

**at least 4 servings per
day; 1 serving = 2 slices
bread, 2 corn tortillas,
⅔ cup flour, 1 cup cereal,
1 cup cooked whole grains**

- Buckwheat
- Corn tortillas
- Gluten-free bread, cereal, pasta, etc. (made without added honey or agave)
- Millet
- Oats, gluten-free

- Quinoa
- Rice
- Starch, potato
- Tapioca

LEGUMES

- Tempeh,
  1 (3½-ounce) slice
- Tofu, firm not silken,
  ⅔ cup

NUTS/SEEDS

2 tablespoons seeds
per day; 1 small handful
of nuts per day

- Brazil nuts
- Chestnuts
- Chia seeds
- Macadamia nuts
- Peanuts
- Pecans
- Pine nuts
- Poppy seeds
- Pumpkin seeds
  (shelled)
- Sesame seeds
- Sunflower seeds
  (shelled)
- Walnuts

HERBS/SPICES/
FLAVORINGS

enjoy unlimited amounts

- Allspice
- Basil

- Bay leaf
- Caraway
- Cardamom
- Chives
- Cilantro/coriander
- Cinnamon
- Cloves
- Cumin
- Curry
- Dill
- Garlic Oil (page 153)
- Ginger
- Marjoram
- Mint
- Mustard
- Nutmeg
- Oregano
- Paprika
- Parsley
- Rosemary
- Sage
- Thyme
- Vanilla

SWEETENERS

limit to 1 serving per day

- Stevia, 2 packets
- Sugar: brown, white,
  1 tablespoon
- Syrup, pure maple,
  2 tablespoons

CONDIMENTS

- Capers
- Chutney
- Horseradish
- Low-FODMAP
  Mayonnaise (page 151)
- Paste: miso, tamarind,
  tomato
- Sauce: fish, oyster,
  soy (gluten-free),
  Worcestershire
- Tahini (sesame seed
  paste), 1 tablespoon
- Vinegar: apple cider,
  red wine, rice, white

MEAT/POULTRY/
EGGS/SEAFOOD

1 to 2 servings per day;
1 serving = 3 ounces

- Any

FATS/OILS

in moderate amounts;
4 tablespoons per day

- Oil: canola, coconut,
  olive, vegetable

OTHER

- Chocolate, dark,
  2 (1-ounce) squares

Moderate-FODMAP Foods to Taste (in small amounts)

DAIRY

amount per day limited to those listed following

- Butter, unsalted, 1 tablespoon
- Cheese: cottage, 2 tablespoons; ricotta, 2 tablespoons
- Half-and-half, 1 tablespoon
- Heavy (whipping) cream, 1 tablespoon

FRUIT

amount per day limited to those listed following

- Avocado, ¼
- Coconut, fresh or flaked, ½ cup

VEGETABLES

amount per day limited to those listed following

- Artichoke hearts, canned, ¼ cup
- Butternut squash, ½ cup
- Celery, 1 stalk
- Pumpkin, 1 cup

GRAINS/CEREALS

amount per day limited to those listed following

- Corn flakes, ½ cup
- Oatmeal: uncooked, not gluten-free, ½ cup; uncooked, quick cooking, 1 cup
- Puffed rice cereal, ½ cup

LEGUMES

amount per day limited to those listed following

- Chickpeas, canned, ¼ cup
- Lentils, canned, scant ½ cup

NUTS/SEEDS

amount per day limited to those listed following

- Almonds, 10
- Hazelnuts, 10

CONDIMENTS

amount per day limited to those listed following

- Hummus, made without garlic, ¼ cup
- Pesto, made without garlic, 1 tablespoon
- Vinegar, balsamic, 2 tablespoons

OTHER

amount per day limited to those listed following

- Chocolate: milk, 1 ounce; white, 1 ounce

Dietary Changes to Reduce IBS Symptoms

And so here we are, ready to explore the nuts and bolts of making dietary changes to help reduce your symptoms. The following tips can help you.

FOLLOW A FODMAP ELIMINATION DIET FOR AT LEAST 30 DAYS

For the next 30 days (or the first 30 days of your low-FODMAP diet plan), eliminate all high-FODMAP foods and stick with the foods listed in the charts on pages 12 and 13, and those in the recipes. If, after 30 days, your symptoms have lessened significantly, you can reintroduce foods to customize the diet to suit your needs. Some people may need longer than 30 days for an elimination diet, so if your symptoms take a little longer to lessen or disappear, consider extending the diet to 45 or even 60 days before reintroducing foods.

AFTER THE ELIMINATION DIET, PERSONALIZE IT

You may have different FODMAP triggers than someone else. Some people may be sensitive to and triggered by all FODMAPs. Others may only be sensitive to fructans and lactose. Therefore, after the initial elimination diet, reintroduce foods to determine your personal triggers.

Do this one food group at a time, starting with a single food. For example, if you'd like to challenge lactose after your 30 days of elimination, try milk with breakfast. Monitor your symptoms. If no symptoms occur by the next day, have a little more. Do this for three or four days. If you are still symptom-free, try other lactose foods, such as cream or cheese. Test for at least a week to determine whether this food will work for you.

You can also do this with other single foods, such as onions. If your symptoms recur, this food is likely one you will always need to avoid. Listen to your body. It will tell you what it needs.

COMPLETELY ELIMINATE FOODS TO WHICH YOU ARE ALLERGIC, SENSITIVE, OR INTOLERANT

You may or may not know what these foods are. To learn what you need to eliminate, again, listen to your body. For example, if you're consuming the foods that are the identified as the most common allergens (see page 4) and still have symptoms, eliminate all of these and reintroduce them one at a time. It's important to note that **if you're concerned about a severe or life-threatening food allergy, work with your doctor.** For food sensitivities and intolerances, consider eliminating these categories:

Alcohol: Avoid drinking alcoholic beverages and do not cook with it.

Corn: It is in everything now, and sometimes in hidden forms. Read labels and you'll be shocked at the number of corn ingredients. Cornstarch. Corn syrup. Caramel coloring. The list goes on. If you are sensitive to corn, familiarize yourself with all the corn-derived ingredients found in processed foods at websites such as LiveCornFree.com.

Gluten and wheat: They are contained in baked goods, breads, cereal, certain condiments, and many other foods.

Histamines: These are commonly found in beer, certain cheeses, champagne, fermented soy products, processed fish, oranges, and wine, among other food items.

Nightshades: This family of foods includes tomatoes, bell peppers, chile peppers, eggplant, potatoes, and goji berries, among others.

Yeast: Yeast is found in beer and wine, as well as in various baked goods such as breads, and in fermented foods.

AVOID FOODS THAT TRIGGER IBS-D

If this is your form of IBS, be aware that some foods that do *not* contain excessive FODMAPs can still make IBS-D worse, according to WebMD. These foods include:

- Caffeine
- Carbonated products
- Chocolate
- Fatty or fried foods
- High-fiber foods
- Fruit juice, in large quantities (as a recipe ingredient in small amounts, fruit juice is fine)

AVOID FOODS THAT TRIGGER IBS-C

If this is your form of IBS, know that some foods may also trigger or worsen IBS-related constipation, according to WebMD. These include:

- Alcohol
- Carbonated products
- Cheese, all types
- Coffee
- Excessive protein
- Processed foods
- Refined (white) grains

IF YOU HAVE GERD OR ACID REFLUX, MAKE GERD FRIENDLY CHANGES

Since GERD can exacerbate IBS symptoms and vice versa, it's important, if you have symptoms, to eat with acid reflux in mind. Try to:

- Avoid alcohol and coffee
- Avoid fried and fatty foods
- Avoid highly acidic foods including vinegar and citrus
- Avoid spicy foods including chilis, black pepper, onions, and garlic
- Eat at least three hours before bedtime
- Eat more ginger in all its forms
- Eat smaller meals
- Don't drink water when you eat

Kitchen Equipment and Pantry List

Even with quick and easy recipes, you need some basic equipment for simplified food prep.

ESSENTIAL EQUIPMENT

There's nothing particularly specialized here—but the following suggestions will keep food prep simple and stress-free.

BLENDER AND/OR FOOD PROCESSOR

I love my food processor and I use it a lot, but I realize not every kitchen has one. If you don't have one, use your blender instead, which you'll definitely need for smoothies and sauces. You can also, in a pinch, use an immersion (stick) blender.

KNIVES

Sharp knives are the most essential tool for any cook. You don't need a big set of fancy expensive knives—just a few decent knives you can keep sharp easily. Sharp knives make chopping safe, quick, and easy. At the very least, you'll need a good chef's or Santoku knife and a paring knife. Other knives are helpful, but optional.

POTS AND PANS

You'll need pots and pans of various sizes and uses, including:

- Baking sheets (one or two)
- Large ovenproof pot with a lid, or a Dutch oven
- Saucepans in small, medium, and large sizes
- Sauté pans or skillets that are nonstick; one should be ovenproof. A well-seasoned 12-inch cast-iron skillet works well. At a minimum, you'll need an ovenproof 12-inch nonstick skillet.

MISCELLANEOUS

As recipes call for measuring, mixing, stirring, scraping, storing, and the usual food prep, make sure you have on hand, and ready to go:

- Measuring cups and spoons
- Small, medium, and large mixing bowls
- Whisks, and scrapers (heat-proof recommended)
- Stirring and peeling utensils
- Food storage containers
- Plastic wrap, aluminum foil, and parchment paper.

OTHER

It's also good to have two cutting boards—one designated for meat (that can be sterilized with bleach, boiling water, or in the dishwasher), and one for vegetables.

NICE-TO-HAVE EQUIPMENT

A 6- to 8-quart slow cooker is the stress-free and super-fast (work-wise) way to prepare your meals. This can be as basic or as fancy as you like, but the benefit is time saved: You just toss in the ingredients in the morning and come home to a kitchen that smells great, a ready-to-eat dinner, and minimal cleanup.

PANTRY STAPLES

Having a well-stocked pantry can help you get on plan and stay on plan. Keep the following items stocked to prepare the recipes, and make it a habit to check your pantry before you go shopping to note items that need to be replenished.

BAKING INGREDIENTS AND FLOURS

- Baking powder
- Baking soda
- Chocolate chips, semi-sweet
- Cocoa powder, unsweetened
- Cornstarch

CANNED AND JARRED ITEMS

- Capers
- Chickpeas
- Lentils
- Olives, black
- Pineapple, in water (unless the recipe specifies juice)
- Pumpkin purée (100 percent pumpkin, *not* pumpkin pie filling)
- Red peppers, roasted
- Tomato paste
- Tomato sauce
- Tomatoes, crushed
- Tuna, water-packed

CONDIMENTS

- Anchovy fillets
- Mustard, Dijon
- Soy sauce or tamari, gluten-free and low-sodium
- Worcestershire sauce

GRAINS

- Bread and buns, gluten-free sandwich
- Bread crumbs, gluten-free
- Flour, buckwheat
- Oats, quick-cooking
- Pasta and spaghetti, gluten-free
- Rice, brown
- Soba noodles
- Tortillas, corn

HERBS AND SPICES

- Cayenne pepper
- Chili powder
- Chinese five-spice powder
- Chinese hot mustard powder
- Cinnamon, ground
- Cumin, ground
- Curry powder
- Italian seasoning, dried
- Nutmeg, ground
- Oregano, dried
- Paprika
- Pepper, black
- Peppercorns
- Red pepper flakes
- Sage, ground
- Sea salt
- Thyme, dried
- Vanilla extract, pure

NUTS AND SEEDS

- Almond butter
- Chia seeds
- Shredded coconut
- Flaxseed
- Macadamia nuts
- Peanut butter, sugar-free, natural
- Pumpkin seeds
- Sesame seeds
- Sunflower seeds
- Tahini

OILS AND VINEGARS

- Cooking spray, nonstick
- Mirin (seasoned rice wine)
- Oil, coconut, extra-virgin
- Oil, olive, extra-virgin
- Oil, sesame
- Vinegar, apple cider
- Vinegar, balsamic
- Vinegar, red wine
- Vinegar, rice

SWEETENERS

- Stevia
- Sugar, granulated white
- Sugar, brown
- Sugar, confectioners'
- Syrup, maple, pure

Low-FODMAP Ingredient Substitutions

REMOVE	REPLACE WITH	NOTES
BARBECUE SAUCE	Homemade Barbecue Sauce	See recipe on page 160.
BROTHS, COMMERCIALLY PREPARED	Low-FODMAP vegetable, poultry, or meat broth	Commercial broths often use garlic and onions. See pages 150 and 152 for recipes.
BUTTERMILK	Lactose-free milk with lemon juice or vinegar added	Combine 1 cup lactose-free milk with 1 tablespoon freshly squeezed lemon juice or vinegar. Let sit for 1 hour.
COW'S MILK	Almond milk, unsweetened, hemp milk, lactose-free milk	Use a 1:1 substitution.
GARLIC	Garlic Oil	See recipe on page 153.
HONEY	Aspartame, maple syrup, stevia	Sweetness varies, so taste as you work.
KETCHUP	¼ cup tomato paste, 2 tablespoons packed brown sugar, 1 tablespoon vinegar, pinch sea salt	Combine the ingredients and simmer for 3 minutes.
LATTE OR CAPPUCCINO	Latte or cappuccino made with unsweetened almond milk	Make a special request from the barista.

Low-FODMAP Ingredient Substitutions

REMOVE	REPLACE WITH	NOTES
ONION	Scallion or leek greens	Exclude the white part.
PASTA	Gluten-free pasta or zucchini noodles	Read labels for other ingredients that might cause an issue.
SAUSAGE, COMMERCIALLY PREPARED	Homemade sausage	Use ground meat combined with herbs like rosemary, thyme, cayenne, and sage.
SOUR CREAM	Lactose-free yogurt	Use plain yogurt.
WHEAT BREAD	Gluten-free bread	My favorites are Canyon Bakehouse and Udi's gluten-free sandwich bread (which may be more widely available).
YOGURT	Dairy-free, lactose-free, or goat's milk	So Delicious makes a tasty and readily available dairy-free yogurt.

Recipe Labels and Tips

Are you ready to start enjoying delicious, easy recipes—and reduced IBS symptoms? In the chapters that follow, you'll find all the recipes you need. Each is labeled and offers tips to help you decide what to cook today and to customize them to your own unique needs.

LABELS

You'll see the following labels on the recipes:

5-Ingredient: These recipes use 5 or fewer main ingredients (excluding oil, herbs, spices, sea salt, pepper, water, or ice) to prepare.

30-Minute: These recipes can be made—start to finish (prep and cooking)— in 30 minutes or fewer.

GERD Friendly: These recipes do not contain any ingredients that will exacerbate acid reflux symptoms. If a recipe is not labeled GERD friendly, or does not include a GERD friendly substitution, avoid the recipe.

Gluten-Free: These recipes do not contain gluten so are safe for people with celiac disease or non-celiac gluten sensitivity.

Low-Carb: These recipes contain 12 or fewer net carbs (total carbs minus fiber) per serving.

Vegan or Vegetarian: Vegan recipes contain no animal ingredients. Vegetarian recipes may contain *eggs or dairy,* but no other animal ingredients.

TIPS

Each recipe will also have one or more tips, using the following designations.

Cooking Tip: Helps clarify or simplify the cooking process.

Ingredient Tip: Offers specific methods for working with ingredients in the recipe or additional information about ingredients.

Substitution Tip: Suggests ingredients you can substitute to make the recipe meet various dietary requirements, such as being GERD friendly or avoiding the Big 8 allergens.

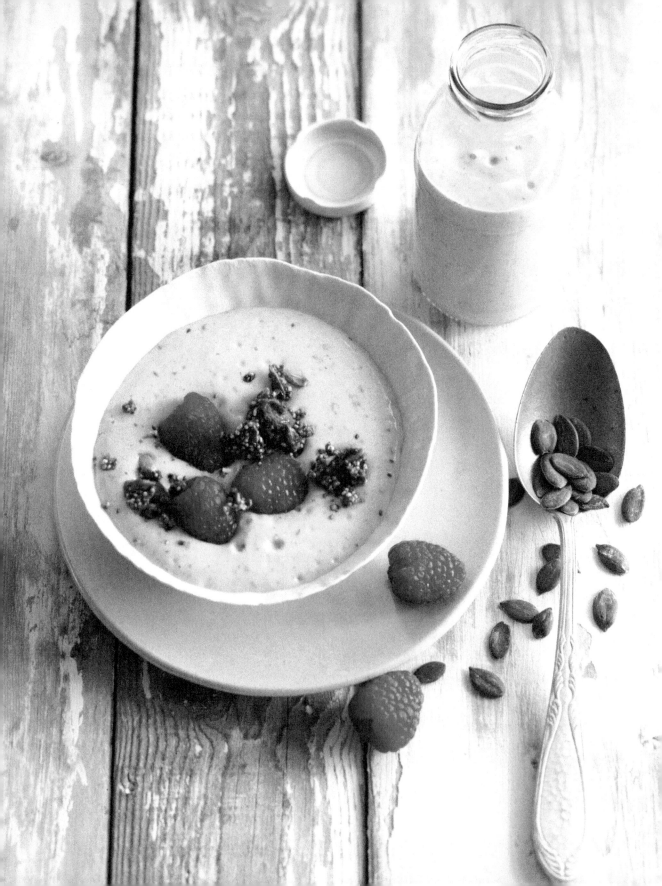

Smoothies *and* Breakfasts

← *Raspberry Smoothie, page 26*

Raspberry Smoothie

5-INGREDIENT | 30-MINUTE | GLUTEN-FREE | LOW-CARB | VEGAN

Prep: 5 minutes
Cook: 0 minutes

2 cups unsweetened
almond milk

1 cup crushed ice

1 cup fresh raspberries

3 tablespoons ground
flaxseed

1 packet stevia (optional)

½ teaspoon vanilla extract

SERVES 2 Start your day with a healthy dose of vitamin C and omega-3 fatty acids in this delicious smoothie. Raspberries are high in antioxidants and vitamin C, while flaxseed is a good source of omega-3 fatty acids. To make this Big 8 Allergen and GERD friendly, see the Tip.

In a blender, combine the almond milk, ice, raspberries, flaxseed, stevia (if using), and vanilla. Blend until smooth.

SUBSTITUTION TIP If you are allergic to tree nuts, replace the almond milk with either unsweetened hemp milk or, if you're *not* allergic or intolerant to dairy products, lactose-free skim milk. To make this GERD friendly, cut your serving size in half.

Per Serving (2 cups) Calories: 177; Total Fat: 9g; Saturated Fat: <1g; Carbohydrates: 20g; Fiber: 7g; Sodium: 181mg; Protein: 5g

PB&J Smoothie

5-INGREDIENT | 30-MINUTE | GLUTEN-FREE | LOW-CARB | VEGAN

SERVES 2 If you love the flavors of peanut butter and jelly, then you'll enjoy this filling smoothie. You can use either fresh or frozen strawberries here. If using frozen berries, make sure they are sugar-free. To make this Big 8 Allergen and GERD friendly, see the Tip.

In a blender, combine the almond milk, strawberries, ice, peanut butter, chia seeds or flaxseed, and stevia (if using). Blend until smooth.

SUBSTITUTION TIP If you are allergic to tree nuts, replace the almond milk with either unsweetened hemp milk or, if you're *not* allergic or intolerant to dairy products, lactose-free skim milk. If you are allergic to peanuts, replace the peanut butter with an equal amount of your favorite unsweetened nut butter. For GERD, reduce the amount of peanut butter by half and cut the serving size in half.

Per Serving (about 2 to 2½ cups) Calories: 328; Total Fat: 25g;
Saturated Fat: 4g; Carbohydrates: 18g; Fiber: 8g; Sodium: 422mg; Protein: 12g

Prep: 5 minutes
Cook: 0 minutes

3 cups unsweetened almond milk

1 cup sliced strawberries, fresh or frozen

1 cup crushed ice

¼ cup sugar-free natural peanut butter

3 tablespoons chia seeds or ground flaxseed

1 packet stevia (optional)

Pineapple-Coconut Smoothie

5-INGREDIENT | 30-MINUTE | GLUTEN-FREE | VEGAN

Prep: 5 minutes
Cook: 0 minutes

2 cups crushed pineapple,
fresh or canned in water
and drained

1 cup canned full-fat
coconut milk

1 cup unsweetened
almond milk

1 cup crushed ice

2 tablespoons chia seeds
or flaxseed

SERVES 2 Coconut milk isn't unlimited on a low-FODMAP food plan, but have only about ½ cup per day, which is the amount in a single serving of this tropical smoothie. You can use either pineapple canned in water (and drained), or fresh pineapple. To make this Big 8 Allergen and GERD friendly, see the Tip.

In a blender, combine the pineapple, coconut milk, almond milk, ice, and chia seeds. Blend until smooth.

SUBSTITUTION TIP If you are allergic to tree nuts, replace the almond milk with an equal amount of hemp milk or, if you're *not* allergic or intolerant to dairy, lactose-free skim milk. If you have GERD, replace the full-fat coconut milk with light coconut milk and reduce the serving size by half.

Per Serving (about 2 to 2½ cups) Calories: 415; Total Fat: 33g;
Saturated Fat: 26g; Carbohydrates: 31g; Fiber: 7g; Sodium: 112mg; Protein: 5g

Sweet Green Smoothie

5-INGREDIENT | 30-MINUTE | GLUTEN-FREE | VEGAN

SERVES 2 This smoothie is a great way to get a healthy serving of nutritious greens to start your day right. While you can use frozen spinach, fresh baby spinach works particularly well here for taste and texture. To make this Big 8 Allergen, GERD, and IBS-D friendly, see the Tip.

In a blender, combine the spinach, almond milk, orange juice, ice, banana, and stevia (if using). Blend until smooth, and sweeten as desired.

SUBSTITUTION TIP If you have GERD or IBS-D, omit the orange juice and replace it with an additional cup of almond milk, and add an extra half banana. If you are allergic to tree nuts, replace the almond milk with an equal amount of unsweetened hemp milk or, if you're *not* allergic or intolerant to dairy, lactose-free skim milk.

Per Serving (about 2 cups) Calories: 159; Total Fat: 4g; Saturated Fat: 0g; Carbohydrates: 30g; Fiber: 4g; Sodium: 217mg; Protein: 4g

Prep: 5 minutes
Cook: 0 minutes

3 cups fresh baby spinach

2 cup unsweetened almond milk

1 cup freshly squeezed orange juice

1 cup crushed ice

1 banana

1 packet stevia (optional), plus more as needed

Melon *and* **Berry Compote**

5-INGREDIENT | 30-MINUTE | GLUTEN-FREE | VEGAN

Prep: 5 minutes
Cook: 0 minutes

2 cups chopped cantaloupe

2 cups fresh blueberries

¼ cup unsweetened
coconut flakes

2 tablespoons flaxseed

SERVES 2 Start your day with this quick and easy fruit salad made from antioxidant-rich berries and sweet, ripe melon. Coconut flakes and flaxseed add a little fat to give the dish some staying power to help you feel full. To make this GERD friendly, see the Tip.

In a medium bowl, gently stir together the cantaloupe, blueberries, coconut flakes, and flaxseed.

INGREDIENT TIP Use in-season berries in this recipe. You can also use strawberries or raspberries. Avoid blackberries and boysenberries, which tend to be too high in FODMAPs.

SUBSTITUTION TIP If you have GERD, omit the coconut flakes to reduce the fat and cut your serving size in half.

Per Serving (about 2 cups) Calories: 196; Total Fat: 5g; Saturated Fat: 2g; Carbohydrates: 36g; Fiber: 7g; Sodium: 29mg; Protein: 4g

Melon *and* Yogurt Parfait

5-INGREDIENT | 30-MINUTE | GLUTEN-FREE | VEGETARIAN

SERVES 2 You can use either coconut milk yogurt or almond milk yogurt here. I like the brand So Delicious, but check your local health food store for your favorite. You can also use lactose-free cow's milk yogurt if you can find it—I suggest Green Valley Organics. With so many different low-FODMAP options, you should be able to find a plain, unsweetened, lactose-free yogurt that works for you. To make this Big 8 Allergen and GERD friendly, see the Tip.

Prep: 5 minutes
Cook: 0 minutes

2 cups chopped honeydew melon, divided

2 cups plain, unsweetened, lactose-free yogurt

¼ cup macadamia nuts, chopped

1. In each of two medium parfait glasses or bowls, place ½ cup honeydew melon.

2. Layer a ½ cup yogurt on top of the melon.

3. Top each with 2 tablespoons macadamia nuts.

4. Repeat with the remaining ingredients.

SUBSTITUTION TIP If you are allergic to tree nuts, replace the macadamia nuts with pumpkin seeds, sunflower seeds, or unsweetened coconut flakes. If you have GERD, reduce the amount of macadamia nuts by half to lower the fat content.

Per Serving (about 2 cups) Calories: 356; Total Fat: 16g; Saturated Fat: 5g; Carbohydrates: 35g; Fiber: 3g; Sodium: 203mg; Protein: 16g

Maple–Brown Sugar Oatmeal

5-INGREDIENT | 30-MINUTE | GERD FRIENDLY | GLUTEN-FREE | VEGETARIAN

Prep: 10 minutes
Cook: 10 minutes

1 cup unsweetened
almond milk

¼ cup packed brown sugar

¼ cup pure maple syrup

1 tablespoon unsalted butter

Pinch sea salt

1 cup quick-cooking oatmeal
(not instant)

SERVES 2 If you are a fan of oatmeal (and want to keep your diet in the FODMAP-friendly range), you can eat up to ½ cup per day. Use quick oats here to save time, but make sure the oats are designated gluten-free. Some oats are processed in the same facilities that process gluten-containing ingredients, and can become cross-contaminated.

1. In a medium saucepan over medium-high heat, heat the almond milk, brown sugar, maple syrup, butter, and salt until it simmers.

2. Stir in the oats. Bring to a boil, stirring frequently.

3. Reduce the heat to medium. Cover and simmer for 5 minutes, until the oatmeal thickens.

INGREDIENT TIP If you have more time, substitute steel-cut oats for an extra fiber boost and richer flavor. Cooking time for steel-cut oats is 10 to 20 minutes depending on how tender you prefer your oats. There are also quick-cooking steel-cut oats available in some markets.

Per Serving (about ½ cup) Calories: 399; Total Fat: 10g; Saturated Fat: 4g; Carbohydrates: 73g; Fiber: 5g; Sodium: 220mg; Protein: 6g

Peanut Butter Pancakes

5-INGREDIENT | 30-MINUTE | GLUTEN-FREE | VEGETARIAN

SERVES 4 Cottage cheese is a dairy product that in small amounts (about ¼ cup per day) won't take you over the top for FODMAP load. Use the full-fat version here, not a low-fat version. These pancakes have a delicious peanut butter flavor and, topped with sliced strawberries, make a delicious PB&J-flavored breakfast. To make this Big 8 Allergen and GERD friendly, see the Tip.

Prep: 5 minutes
Cook: 10 minutes

4 eggs

1 cup creamy sugar-free natural peanut butter

¼ cup cottage cheese

2 tablespoons pure maple syrup

1 teaspoon vanilla extract

1 cup sliced fresh strawberries

Nonstick cooking spray

1. Heat a skillet over medium-high heat.

2. In a blender or food processor, combine the eggs, peanut butter, cottage cheese, maple syrup, and vanilla. Blend until smooth.

3. In 2-tablespoon amounts, pour the batter onto the heated skillet, 3 pancakes at a time, leaving room for each to spread. Cook for 2 to 3 minutes, until bubbles form on the surface. Flip each pancake and cook the other side for 2 to 3 minutes until browned at the edges.

4. Transfer to a plate, and serve topped with the sliced strawberries.

SUBSTITUTION TIP If you are allergic or intolerant to dairy products, replace the cottage cheese with an unsweetened plain nut yogurt, such as almond milk yogurt or coconut milk yogurt. To make this GERD friendly, reduce the serving size by half and use low-fat or fat-free cottage cheese.

Per Serving (3 pancakes) Calories: 495; Total Fat: 37g; Saturated Fat: 8g; Carbohydrates: 23g; Fiber: 5g; Sodium: 417mg; Protein: 24g

Pumpkin Pie Pancakes

5-INGREDIENT | 30-MINUTE | GERD FRIENDLY | GLUTEN-FREE | LOW-CARB | VEGETARIAN

Prep: 5 minutes
Cook: 10 minutes

1 cup pumpkin purée

4 eggs, beaten

1 tablespoon ground flaxseed

1 tablespoon buckwheat flour

1 teaspoon baking powder

1 teaspoon pumpkin pie spice

Pinch sea salt

Nonstick cooking spray

SERVES 4 The sweet spices of these pumpkin pancakes will take you instantly to the holidays, and the flavors blend well with pure maple syrup if you want to use that as a topping. This recipe is quick and easy—perfect for a Saturday morning breakfast with the family.

1. In a small bowl, whisk the pumpkin purée and eggs until well mixed.

2. In a medium bowl, whisk the flaxseed, buckwheat flour, baking powder, pumpkin pie spice, and salt.

3. Fold the wet ingredients into the dry ingredients until combined.

4. Spray a large nonstick skillet with cooking spray and place it over medium-high heat.

5. Spoon the batter in scant ¼-cup amounts onto the heated skillet. With the back of a spoon, spread the batter thin. Cook for about 3 minutes, until bubbles form on the top. Flip and cook for about 3 minutes more, until browned on the other side.

INGREDIENT TIP You may have heard on social media that most canned pumpkin isn't pumpkin at all, but actually squash. This is not true. If the can lists 100 percent pumpkin, it contains pumpkin—so look for pumpkin purée that says 100 percent pumpkin on the label.

Per Serving (3 pancakes) Calories: 102; Total Fat: 5g; Saturated Fat: 2g; Carbohydrates: 8g; Fiber: 3g; Sodium: 105mg; Protein: 7g

French Toast

5-INGREDIENT | 30-MINUTE | GERD FRIENDLY | GLUTEN-FREE | LOW-CARB | VEGETARIAN

SERVES 2 It's easy to make a basic delicious low-FODMAP French toast, and you can customize this version with different spices or extracts to pump up the flavor. Serve with pure maple syrup or topped with a sprinkling of confectioners' sugar.

1. In a medium bowl, whisk together the eggs, almond milk, vanilla, orange zest, stevia, and nutmeg.

2. Soak the bread slices in the mixture for about 5 minutes.

3. Spray a large nonstick skillet with cooking spray and place it over medium-high heat.

4. Add the soaked bread. Cook for about 5 minutes, until browned on one side. Flip and cook for 3 to 4 more minutes on the other side.

INGREDIENT TIP Look for gluten-free bread in the freezer section of your grocery store.

Per Serving (2 slices) Calories: 206; Total Fat: 12g; Saturated Fat: 3g; Carbohydrates: 12g; Fiber: 1g; Sodium: 336mg; Protein: 13g

Prep: 5 minutes
Rest: 5 minutes
Cook: 10 minutes

4 eggs, beaten

1 cup unsweetened almond milk

1 teaspoon vanilla extract

1 teaspoon grated orange zest

1 packet stevia

½ teaspoon ground nutmeg

4 gluten-free bread slices

Nonstick cooking spray

Banana Toast

5-INGREDIENT | 30-MINUTE | GERD FRIENDLY | GLUTEN-FREE | VEGETARIAN

Prep: 5 minutes
Cook: 5 minutes

4 gluten-free sandwich bread slices

1 ripe banana

½ teaspoon ground cinnamon

SERVES 2 Nothing is easier than banana toast. With just three ingredients and a cooking time that lasts as long as it takes your toaster to toast bread, you can be out the door quickly in the morning with this portable and tasty breakfast.

1. Toast the bread to your desired doneness.

2. In a small bowl, mash the banana with the cinnamon and spread it on the toast.

COOKING TIP Ripe or very ripe bananas work best here because they mash most easily, so this is a great way to use up those overripe bananas. Get creative: Mix sunflower seeds or pepitas (hulled pumpkin seeds) into the mashed banana for a bit of crunch.

Per Serving (2 slices) Calories: 102; Total Fat: <1g; Saturated Fat: 0g; Carbohydrates: 23g; Fiber: 2g; Sodium: 123mg; Protein: 2g

Fried Eggs *with* Potato Hash

5-INGREDIENT | GLUTEN-FREE | VEGETARIAN

SERVES 2 If you have a little extra time in the morning, start your day with this simple hash topped with over-easy fried eggs. The egg yolks remain soft and burst open when you cut into them to coat the crispy caramelized potatoes. Good morning! To make this GERD friendly, see the Tip.

Prep: 10 minutes
Cook: 26 minutes

2 tablespoons Garlic Oil (page 153), plus more as needed

2 russet potatoes, cut into ½-inch cubes

3 scallions, green parts only, chopped

½ teaspoon sea salt, plus more for seasoning the eggs

¼ teaspoon freshly ground black pepper, plus more for seasoning the eggs

4 eggs

1. In a large skillet over medium-high heat, heat the garlic oil until it shimmers.

2. Add the potatoes. Cook for about 20 minutes, stirring occasionally, until soft and browned.

3. Add the scallions, salt, and pepper. Cook for 1 minute more, stirring frequently. Spoon the potatoes onto two plates.

4. Return the skillet to medium heat. If the pan is dry, add a little more garlic oil and swirl it to coat the skillet (see Tip).

5. Carefully crack the eggs into the skillet and season them with a pinch of salt and pepper. Cook undisturbed for 3 to 4 minutes, until the whites solidify.

6. Turn off the heat and carefully flip the eggs so you do not break the yolk. Leave the eggs in the hot pan for 60 to 90 seconds until the surface is cooked but the yolks remain runny.

7. Serve the potatoes topped with the eggs.

SUBSTITUTION TIP To make this GERD friendly, replace the garlic oil with 1 tablespoon olive oil. Omit the black pepper.

Per Serving (2 eggs, 1 cup potatoes) Calories: 401; Total Fat: 23g; Saturated Fat: 5g; Carbohydrates: 36g; Fiber: 6g; Sodium: 608mg; Protein: 15g

Tofu Breakfast Scramble

5-INGREDIENT | 30-MINUTE | GERD FRIENDLY | GLUTEN-FREE | VEGAN

Prep: 10 minutes
Cook: 8 minutes

2 tablespoons Garlic Oil
(page 153)

1⅓ cups firm tofu, cut into
1-inch pieces

1 red bell pepper, chopped

1 medium zucchini, chopped

½ teaspoon sea salt

¼ teaspoon freshly ground
black pepper

SERVES 2 Although tofu is a legume, you can avoid going over your FODMAP load by limiting the amount you eat to ⅔ cup per serving. To stretch that amount while still benefiting from tofu as a good source of protein, this scramble adds veggies for color, flavor, and nutrition. To make this Big 8 Allergen friendly, see the Tip.

1. In a large skillet over medium-high heat, heat the garlic oil until it shimmers.

2. Add the tofu, bell pepper, zucchini, salt, and pepper. Cook for about 6 minutes, stirring occasionally, until the vegetables soften and begin to brown slightly.

INGREDIENT TIP Tofu can be a bit watery. If you'd like to make it less so, place the tofu in a colander in the sink and put a plate on top of it with a heavy can weighing down the plate. Allow it to compress for about 10 minutes so the water runs off before slicing.

SUBSTITUTION TIP If you are allergic to soy, replace the tofu with 4 eggs (in which case, this recipe will not suit vegans). Add the eggs directly to the veggies after they have cooked, scrambling them for about 3 minutes.

Per Serving (2 cups) Calories: 273; Total Fat: 23g; Saturated Fat: 5g; Carbohydrates: 36g; Fiber: 6g; Sodium: 608mg; Protein: 15g

Easy Breakfast Sausage

5-INGREDIENT | 30-MINUTE | GLUTEN-FREE | LOW-CARB

SERVES 4 Mix up a batch of this easy breakfast sausage to serve with eggs, potatoes, or as part of a Sausage and Egg Omelet (page 40). You can also use different types of ground meat to vary the fat content—something you'll want to do if you have GERD (see Tip).

Prep: 10 minutes
Cook: 8 minutes

1 pound ground pork

1 teaspoon ground sage

½ teaspoon sea salt

⅛ teaspoon red pepper flakes

⅛ teaspoon freshly ground black pepper

Nonstick cooking spray

1. In a large bowl, mix the pork, sage, salt, red pepper flakes, and pepper. Form the mixture into 8 patties.

2. Spray a large nonstick skillet with cooking spray and place it over medium-high heat.

3. Add the sausage patties and cook for about 4 minutes per side, until browned on both sides.

SUBSTITUTION TIP For GERD, use ground turkey breast and reduce the serving size to 1 patty.

Per Serving (2 patties) Calories: 163; Total Fat: 4g; Saturated Fat: 1g; Carbohydrates: <1g; Fiber: 0g; Sodium: 299mg; Protein: 30g

Sausage *and* Egg Omelet

5-INGREDIENT | 30-MINUTE | GLUTEN-FREE | LOW-CARB

Prep: 10 minutes
Cook: 8 minutes

6 eggs, beaten

¼ cup unsweetened
almond milk

¼ teaspoon sea salt

¼ teaspoon freshly ground
black pepper

Nonstick cooking spray

½ pound cooked, hot Easy
Breakfast Sausage (page 39),
cut into small pieces

¼ cup grated Cheddar cheese

SERVES 2 This easy omelet uses Easy Breakfast Sausage (page 39) as an ingredient—if you have time, make it today, or use up leftover cooked patties. You can save more time by buying already grated cheese. You'll need your pan to be well oiled to flip the omelet. Alternatively, you can just scramble all the ingredients together and add the cheese at the end. To make this GERD and IBS-C friendly, see the Tip.

1. In a large bowl, whisk the eggs, almond milk, salt, and pepper.

2. Spray a large nonstick skillet with cooking spray and place it over medium-high heat.

3. Add the eggs and cook for about 3 minutes until they start to solidify. With a spatula, gently pull the cooked eggs away from the edge of the pan. Tilt the pan so any uncooked egg flows into the spaces you've created. Continue cooking the eggs for about 3 minutes more.

4. Spread the sausage and cheese over half the omelet. Fold the other side over the filling. Cook for 1 to 2 minutes more to melt the cheese.

SUBSTITUTION TIP For a GERD friendly version, use ground turkey breast sausage and omit the cheese. If you have IBS-C, omit the cheese.

Per Serving (½ omelet) Calories: 580; Total Fat: 36g; Saturated Fat: 17g; Carbohydrates: 2g; Fiber: 0g; Sodium: 470mg; Protein: 60g

Tropical Fruit Salad

5-INGREDIENT | 30-MINUTE | GERD FRIENDLY | GLUTEN-FREE | VEGAN

SERVES 4 Tropical fruits tend to be relatively low in FODMAPS (with the exception of mangos), so they are a delicious way to add sweet, exotic flavors to your meals. This light, easy tropical salad is delicious on its own, for breakfast, or as a side dish for a light meal, such as fish or shellfish.

In a medium bowl, gently stir together the bananas, papaya, pineapple chunks, and coconut.

INGREDIENT TIP Only buy canned pineapple that is packed in its own juice or in water, not syrup. Also, if you can't find fresh papaya, replace it with 1 cup cantaloupe.

Per Serving (about 1 cup) Calories: 116; Total Fat: 1g; Saturated Fat: <1g; Carbohydrates: 28g; Fiber: 4g; Sodium: 8m; Protein: 1g

Prep: 10 minutes
Cook: 0 minutes

2 bananas, sliced

1 papaya, peeled, seeded, and cut into bite-size cubes

1 cup pineapple chunks, fresh or canned, drained

2 tablespoons unsweetened shredded coconut

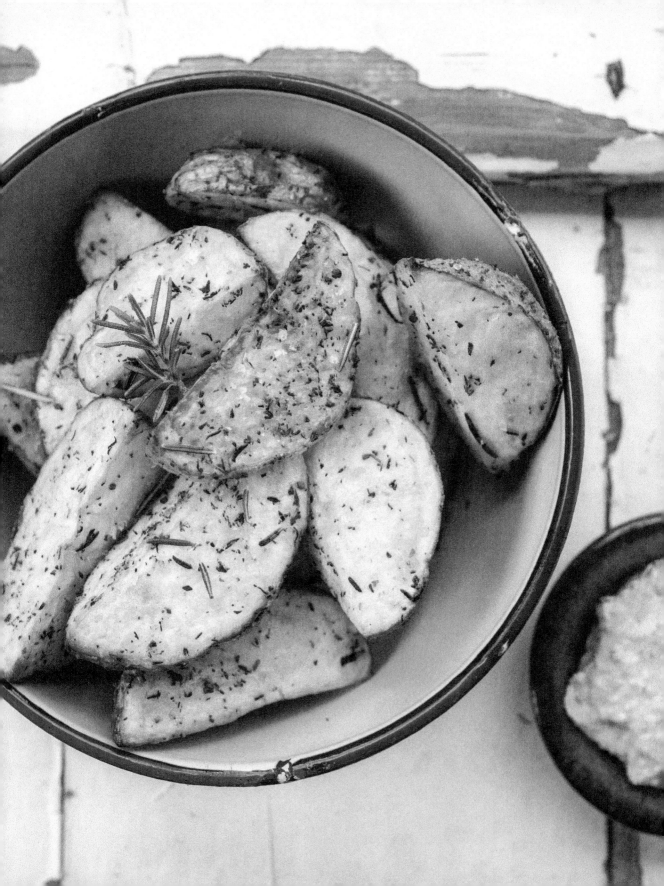

THREE

Salads *and* Sides

← *Roasted Potato Wedges, page 55*

Chopped Italian Salad

5-INGREDIENT | 30-MINUTE | GLUTEN-FREE | LOW-CARB | VEGAN

Prep: 10 minutes
Cook: 0 minutes

4 cups chopped romaine lettuce

8 cherry tomatoes, halved

1 medium zucchini, chopped

1 cup black olives, halved

¼ cup Italian Balsamic Vinaigrette (page 156)

SERVES 4 Chopped salads make a delicious side dish for pasta or, if you add some protein, they can be tasty main dishes. To make this protein rich and GERD friendly, see the Tip.

1. In a medium bowl, combine the lettuce, tomatoes, zucchini, and olives.

2. Add the vinaigrette and toss to coat.

SUBSTITUTION TIP Add 6 ounces of precooked chopped chicken breast chunks to make this side salad into a well-rounded meal. To make it GERD friendly, omit the tomatoes.

Per Serving (about 1½ cups) Calories: 158; Total Fat: 10g; Saturated Fat: 2g; Carbohydrates: 16g; Fiber: 5g; Sodium: 433mg; Protein: 3g

Warm Spinach Salad

5-INGREDIENT | 30-MINUTE | GLUTEN-FREE | LOW-CARB

SERVES 4 A simple spinach salad becomes delectable with a warm dressing made from bacon fat and vinegar. The warm dressing gently wilts the raw spinach and adds rich flavor.

Prep: 10 minutes
Cook: 8 minutes

6 cups fresh baby spinach

4 bacon slices, chopped

4 scallions, green parts only, finely chopped

¼ cup red wine vinegar

½ teaspoon sea salt

¼ teaspoon freshly ground black pepper

1. Place the spinach in a large bowl and refrigerate until ready to serve.

2. In a large skillet over medium-high heat, cook the bacon for about 5 minutes, stirring occasionally, until browned. With a slotted spoon, transfer the bacon to a plate and set it aside. Leave the fat in the pan. Return the skillet to medium-high heat.

3. Stir the scallions, vinegar, salt, and pepper into the bacon fat. Bring to a simmer. Reduce the heat to low and cook the dressing for 3 to 5 minutes, stirring occasionally, until it thickens.

4. Pour the warm dressing over the spinach and gently toss to coat and lightly wilt the leaves.

INGREDIENT TIP This recipe works best when the spinach is very dry. To do this, after washing the spinach in a colander, pat the leaves dry between paper towels or spin them in a salad spinner to remove all moisture.

Per Serving (about 1½ cups) Calories: 172; Total Fat: 12g; Saturated Fat: 4g; Carbohydrates: 3g; Fiber: 1g; Sodium: 928mg; Protein: 12g

Caprese Salad

5-INGREDIENT | 30-MINUTE | GLUTEN-FREE | VEGETARIAN

Prep: 10 minutes
Cook: 0 minutes

2 cups torn romaine lettuce

20 cherry tomatoes, quartered

¼ cup loosely packed fresh basil leaves, chopped

4 ounces mozzarella cheese, chopped

¼ cup Italian Basil Vinaigrette (page 155)

SERVES 4 A traditional Caprese salad has layers of tomatoes, whole basil leaves, and fresh mozzarella cheese. This is a chopped version, but the flavors are just as enticing. The addition of salad greens makes the salad a bit heartier. To make this GERD and IBS-C friendly, see the Tip.

1. In a large bowl, combine the lettuce, tomatoes, basil, and cheese.

2. Add the vinaigrette and toss to coat.

SUBSTITUTION TIP To make this GERD friendly, replace the cherry tomatoes with ½ cup black olives. If you have IBS-C, avoid this recipe.

Per Serving (about 1½ cups) Calories: 265; Total Fat: 14g; Saturated Fat: 5g; Carbohydrates: 26g; Fiber: 8g; Sodium: 202mg; Protein: 14g

Easy Fruit Salad

5-INGREDIENT | 30-MINUTE | GLUTEN-FREE | VEGETARIAN

SERVES 4 A salad made of simple fruits is a beautiful thing—sweet, flavorful, and packed with nutrition. This recipe uses all low-FODMAP fruits so it won't exceed your FODMAP load, and it packs easily for a quick meal on the go. To make this GERD friendly, see the Tip.

In a large bowl, gently stir together the clementines, strawberries, blueberries, and bananas.

SUBSTITUTION TIP To make this a GERD friendly dish, replace the clementines with 2 cups chopped cantaloupe.

Per Serving (about 1 cup) Calories: 133; Total Fat: <1g; Saturated Fat: 0g; Carbohydrates: 34g; Fiber: 5g; Sodium: 2mg; Protein: 2g

Prep: 10 minutes
Cook: 0 minutes

6 clementines, sectioned

2 cups sliced fresh strawberries

1 pint fresh blueberries

2 bananas, sliced

Roasted Root Vegetable Salad

5-INGREDIENT | GLUTEN-FREE | VEGAN

Prep: 10 minutes
Cook: 45 minutes

4 carrots, cut into
½-inch pieces

4 red potatoes, cut into
½-inch cubes

1 fennel bulb, cut into
½-inch pieces

2 tablespoons extra-virgin
olive oil

¼ cup Lemon-Dill Vinaigrette
(page 157)

SERVES 4 Roasting root veggies gives them a rich caramelized flavor that brings a lot to this simple salad. While it takes a while to roast the veggies, most of that time is inactive, and your total work time is only about 10 minutes.

1. Preheat the oven to 400°F.

2. Line two baking sheets with parchment paper.

3. In a large bowl, toss the carrots, potatoes, and fennel with the olive oil. Divide the vegetables between the two prepared sheets and spread in a single layer.

4. Roast for about 45 minutes, until the veggies are browned, stirring occasionally, rotating the pans and switching racks halfway through cooking. Cool slightly.

5. Drizzle the vinaigrette over the vegetables and toss to coat.

INGREDIENT TIP Fennel looks a lot like celery. The part you want here is the bulb—the bottom part, not the celery-looking stalks, which you can save for another use. Use a sharp knife to cut out the core of the root by halving the root lengthwise and trimming out the hard core.

Per Serving (about 1½ cups) Calories: 342; Total Fat: 15g; Saturated Fat: 3g; Carbohydrates: 49g; Fiber: 8g; Sodium: 85mg; Protein: 6g

Quick Creamy Coleslaw

30-MINUTE | GLUTEN-FREE | LOW-CARB | VEGETARIAN

SERVES 4 Creamy coleslaw makes a tasty side dish for all kinds of proteins, such as Chicken Tenders (page 115) or Breaded Fish Fillets with Spicy Pepper Relish (page 102). To make this protein rich and GERD friendly, see the Tip.

Prep: 15 minutes
Cook: 0 minutes

1 head green cabbage, shredded, or 1 (8-ounce) package preshredded green cabbage

4 scallions, green parts only, chopped

2 carrots, grated

¼ cup Low-FODMAP Mayonnaise (page 151)

1 tablespoon apple cider vinegar

¼ teaspoon ground mustard

½ teaspoon sea salt

¼ teaspoon freshly ground black pepper

1. In a large bowl, combine the cabbage, scallions, and carrots.

2. In a small bowl, whisk together the mayonnaise, vinegar, mustard, salt, and pepper. Add the sauce to the coleslaw and toss to coat.

SUBSTITUTION TIP To make this GERD friendly, omit the black pepper and vinegar, and replace with the grated zest of 1 orange. You can also add 3 ounces (per serving) of cooked, shredded chicken to make this slaw into a complete meal.

Per Serving (about 1 cup) Calories: 121; Total Fat: 5g; Saturated Fat: <1g; Carbohydrates: 18g; Fiber: 6g; Sodium: 394mg; Protein: 3g

Cucumber *and* Sesame Salad

5-INGREDIENT | 30-MINUTE | GLUTEN-FREE | LOW-CARB | VEGAN

Prep: 10 minutes
Cook: 0 minutes

4 medium cucumbers, peeled and chopped

6 scallions, green parts only, chopped

1 tablespoon sesame seeds

1 teaspoon sesame oil

¼ cup Cilantro-Lime Vinaigrette (page 154)

SERVES 4 Rich, nutty sesame oil serves as a tasty counterpoint to the fresh flavor of the cucumbers in this quick and tasty salad. If you have a spiralizer, it's fun to turn the cucumbers into noodle shapes, but chopping works equally well. To make this GERD friendly, see the Tip.

1. In a large bowl, combine the cucumbers, scallions, and sesame seeds.

2. In a small bowl, whisk together the sesame oil and vinaigrette. Add the dressing to the cucumber mix and toss to coat.

SUBSTITUTION TIP To make this GERD friendly, replace the cucumbers with zucchini.

Per Serving (about 1 cup) Calories: 145; Total Fat: 10g; Saturated Fat: 2g; Carbohydrates: 14g; Fiber: 2g; Sodium: 10mg; Protein: 3g

Kale *and* Red Bell Pepper Salad

5-INGREDIENT | 30-MINUTE | GLUTEN-FREE | LOW-CARB | VEGAN

SERVES 4 Kale is high in antioxidants, while red bell pepper adds color, nutrients, and a sweet crunch to this tasty salad. Serve this as a side dish, or add 3 ounces cooked shrimp (per serving) for a tasty main course. To make this GERD friendly, see the Tip.

1. In a large bowl, combine the kale, bell pepper, and pepitas.
2. Add the vinaigrette and toss to coat.

SUBSTITUTION TIP To make this GERD friendly, replace the red bell peppers with ½ cup black or green olives, halved.

Per Serving (about 1 cup) Calories: 149; Total Fat: 10g; Saturated Fat: 2g; Carbohydrates: 12g; Fiber: 2g; Sodium: 151mg; Protein: 4g

Prep: 10 minutes
Cook: 0 minutes

4 cups stemmed, chopped kale, or 1 (9-ounce) bag kale salad

1 red bell pepper, stemmed, seeded, and chopped

¼ cup pepitas (hulled pumpkin seeds)

¼ cup Balsamic Vinaigrette (page 156)

Sesame-Broccoli Stir-Fry

5-INGREDIENT | 30-MINUTE | GERD FRIENDLY | GLUTEN-FREE | LOW-CARB | VEGAN

Prep: 10 minutes
Cook: 10 minutes

2 tablespoons extra-virgin olive oil

2 cups broccoli florets

2 tablespoons gluten-free soy sauce

½ teaspoon sesame oil

2 tablespoons sesame seeds

SERVES 4 Stir-frying broccoli until it is crisp-tender keeps its flavor and nutrients intact. The rich sesame oil adds a deep flavor to this dish. This is a great side for steamed fish or roasted chicken. If you'd like to make a complete meal of it, add 3 ounces cooked animal protein (per serving). Note that broccoli at a ½-cup serving size won't create an overabundant FODMAP load; however, a full cup is a bit high, so watch out how much broccoli you eat in a day.

1. In a large skillet over medium-high heat, heat the olive oil until it shimmers.

2. Add the broccoli. Cook for about 6 minutes, stirring occasionally, until crisp-tender.

3. Stir in the soy sauce and sesame oil. Bring to a simmer. Reduce the heat to medium and cook for 3 minutes, stirring.

4. Toss with the sesame seeds before serving.

INGREDIENT TIP To save time, buy broccoli already separated into florets. To separate them yourself, trim away the heavy stem and then snap off the small individual florets. Cut them into smaller pieces if needed.

Per Serving (about ½ cup) Calories: 111; Total Fat: 10g; Saturated Fat: 1g; Carbohydrates: 5g; Fiber: 2g; Sodium: 466mg; Protein: 3g

Orange-Maple Glazed Carrots

5-INGREDIENT | 30-MINUTE | GLUTEN-FREE | LOW-CARB | VEGAN

SERVES 4 Carrots are especially low in FODMAPs, so they make a great side or snack that won't significantly affect your FODMAP load. Here, baby carrots make prep time super quick and easy. Be sure to purchase pure maple syrup, not maple-flavored syrup, which may be made with corn syrup. Maple syrup, at about 1 tablespoon per day, won't increase your FODMAP load. To make this GERD friendly, see the Tip.

Prep: 5 minutes
Cook: 20 minutes

2 tablespoons pure maple syrup

1 tablespoon extra-virgin olive oil

Juice of 1 orange

Zest of 1 orange

½ teaspoon sea salt

¼ teaspoon freshly ground black pepper

2 cups baby carrots

1. Preheat the oven to 400°F.

2. Line a baking sheet with parchment paper and set it aside.

3. In a medium bowl, whisk together the maple syrup, olive oil, orange juice, orange zest, salt, and pepper.

4. Add the carrots and toss to coat.

5. Spread the carrots in a single layer on the prepared sheet. Roast for 20 minutes, or until browned.

SUBSTITUTION TIP To make this GERD friendly, omit the orange juice (but keep the orange zest) and add 2 tablespoons water. The zest will flavor the carrots and shouldn't aggravate your GERD.

Per Serving (about ½ cup) Calories: 101; Total Fat: 4g; Saturated Fat: <1g; Carbohydrates: 17g; Fiber: 2g; Sodium: 298mg; Protein: 1g

Mashed Potatoes

5-INGREDIENT | 30-MINUTE | GLUTEN-FREE | VEGETARIAN

Prep: 10 minutes
Cook: 10 minutes

4 russet potatoes, peeled and cut into 1-inch cubes

2 tablespoons unsalted butter

¼ cup unsweetened almond milk

½ teaspoon sea salt

¼ teaspoon freshly ground black pepper

SERVES 4 This classic comfort food is tasty by itself as a snack, makes a perfect side dish for Quick Meatloaf Patties (page 124) or other animal proteins, and is quick and easy to prepare. To make this GERD friendly, see the Tip.

1. In a large pot over medium-high heat, combine the potatoes with enough water to cover. Bring to a boil and cook for 10 to 15 minutes, until soft. Drain and return the potatoes to the pot.

2. Add the butter, almond milk, salt, and pepper. With a potato masher, mash until smooth.

SUBSTITUTION TIP To make this GERD friendly, reduce the butter to 1 tablespoon and omit the black pepper. If you are allergic to tree nuts, replace the almond milk with hemp milk or lactose-free milk.

Per Serving (about ½ cup) Calories: 233; Total Fat: 10g; Saturated Fat: 7g; Carbohydrates: 34g; Fiber: 6g; Sodium: 290mg; Protein: 4g

Roasted Potato Wedges

5-INGREDIENT | GLUTEN-FREE | LOW-CARB | VEGAN

SERVES 4 There's something about the pairing of potatoes and fragrant rosemary that is especially satisfying and delicious. While roasting the potatoes takes about 30 minutes, most of your time is inactive, just waiting for them to cook. To make this GERD friendly, see the Tip.

Prep: 10 minutes
Cook: 30 minutes

1 pound Yukon Gold potatoes, quartered lengthwise

2 tablespoons Garlic Oil (page 153)

1 tablespoon chopped fresh rosemary leaves

½ teaspoon sea salt

¼ teaspoon freshly ground black pepper

1. Preheat the oven to 425°F.

2. In a large bowl, toss the potatoes with the garlic oil, rosemary, salt, and pepper. Divide them between two baking sheets and spread into a single layer.

3. Bake for about 30 minutes until the potatoes are browned. Stir them once or twice and rotate the pans (switching racks) halfway through cooking.

SUBSTITUTION TIP To make this GERD friendly, omit the garlic oil and black pepper. Instead, use 1 tablespoon olive oil.

Per Serving (about ½ cup) Calories: 143; Total Fat: 7g; Saturated Fat: 1g; Carbohydrates: 19g; Fiber: 2g; Sodium: 241mg; Protein: 2g

Parmesan Baked Zucchini

5-INGREDIENT | 30-MINUTE | LOW-CARB | GLUTEN-FREE | VEGETARIAN

Prep: 10 minutes
Cook: 17 minutes

4 zucchini, quartered lengthwise

2 tablespoons Garlic Oil (page 153)

¼ cup freshly grated Parmesan cheese

½ teaspoon chopped fresh thyme leaves

½ teaspoon sea salt

¼ teaspoon freshly ground black pepper

SERVES 4 These delightful zucchini bites are loaded with flavor, and the Parmesan cheese adds a nice piquancy to zucchini's mild taste. Broiling at the end helps crisp the zucchini, so it's almost like eating a delicious and nutritious French fry. To make this GERD, IBS-C, and Big 8 Allergen friendly, see the Tip.

1. Preheat the oven to 350°F.

2. In a large bowl, toss together the zucchini, garlic oil, cheese, thyme, salt, and pepper. Place the zucchini, skin-side down, in a single layer on a rimmed baking sheet.

3. Bake for about 15 minutes, until soft.

4. Set the oven to broil.

5. Broil the zucchini for 2 to 3 minutes, until browned and crisp.

SUBSTITUTION TIP If you have IBS-C or are allergic or intolerant to dairy products, omit the cheese and add ½ teaspoon dried oregano to the spice blend. To make this GERD friendly, omit the black pepper and garlic oil and use 1 tablespoon olive oil instead.

Per Serving (1 zucchini) Calories: 183; Total Fat: 13g; Saturated Fat: 5g; Carbohydrates: 8g; Fiber: 2g; Sodium: 517mg; Protein: 12g

Easy Rice Pilaf

5-INGREDIENT | 30-MINUTE | GLUTEN-FREE | VEGAN

SERVES 4 Using precooked rice (look for it in the rice aisle or freezer section of the grocery store) makes this recipe come together quickly. The recipe includes pine nuts, which won't tip your FODMAP load over the top at a 1-tablespoon serving size. Rice, at up to about 1 cup per day, will also help keep FODMAPs low. To make this GERD friendly, see the Substitution Tip.

Prep: 10 minutes
Cook: 10 minutes

2 tablespoons extra-virgin olive oil

6 scallions, green parts only, chopped

2 carrots, chopped

2 cups cooked brown rice

¼ cup pine nuts

½ teaspoon sea salt

⅛ teaspoon freshly ground black pepper

¼ cup chopped fresh parsley leaves

1. In a large skillet over medium-high heat, heat the olive oil until it shimmers.

2. Add the scallions and carrots. Cook for about 4 minutes, stirring occasionally.

3. Stir in the brown rice, pine nuts, salt, and pepper. Cook for about 5 minutes more, stirring occasionally, until the rice is warm.

4. Stir in the parsley just before serving.

INGREDIENT TIP If you can't find precooked brown rice, cook a big batch on a weekend and then freeze it in 1-cup portions. It will keep in a zip-top bag in the freezer for up to 12 months.

SUBSTITUTION TIP To make this GERD friendly, reduce the olive oil to 1 tablespoon and omit the black pepper.

Per Serving (about ½ cup) Calories: 307; Total Fat: 13g; Saturated Fat: 2g; Carbohydrates: 43g; Fiber: 2g; Sodium: 263mg; Protein: 5g

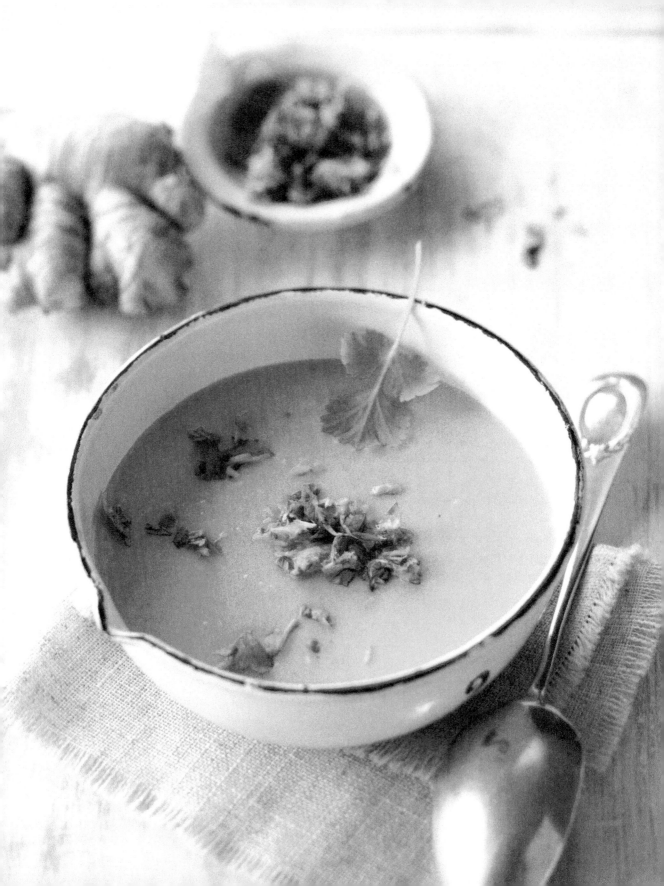

Soups *and* Sandwiches

← *Carrot and Ginger Soup, page 61*

Shrimp Chowder

30-MINUTE | GLUTEN-FREE

Prep: 10 minutes
Cook: 20 minutes

2 tablespoons Garlic Oil
(page 153)

6 scallions, green parts only,
chopped

1 fennel bulb, chopped

2 carrots, chopped

7 cups Low-FODMAP
Poultry Broth (page 152)

8 baby red potatoes,
quartered

½ teaspoon sea salt

¼ teaspoon freshly ground
black pepper

12 ounces medium shrimp,
peeled, deveined, and
tails removed

1 cup unsweetened
almond milk

2 tablespoons cornstarch

2 tablespoons chopped
fennel fronds

SERVES 4 This tasty, creamy chowder doesn't take long to make. If you prefer a different type of seafood, replace the shrimp with an equal amount of clams, crabmeat, or fish. To make this GERD friendly, see the Tip.

1. In a large pot over medium-high, heat the garlic oil until it shimmers.

2. Add the scallions, fennel bulb, and carrots. Cook for about 3 minutes, stirring occasionally, until soft.

3. Stir in the broth, potatoes, salt, and pepper. Simmer for 10 minutes, until the potatoes are tender.

4. Add the shrimp. Cook for 5 minutes more.

5. In a small bowl, whisk the almond milk and cornstarch into a slurry. Stir this mixture into the soup in a thin stream. Simmer the soup for about 2 minutes more until it thickens.

6. Stir in the fennel fronds.

INGREDIENT TIP Look for uncooked deveined shrimp with tails removed in the freezer section of your grocery store. This will save the time it takes to prep the shrimp.

SUBSTITUTION TIP To make this GERD friendly, replace the garlic oil with 2 tablespoons olive oil. Omit the scallions and pepper.

Per Serving (2 cups) Calories: 325; Total Fat: 10g; Saturated Fat: 2g; Carbohydrates: 33g; Fiber: 5g; Sodium: 671mg; Protein: 27g

Carrot *and* Ginger Soup

5-INGREDIENT | 30-MINUTE | GERD FRIENDLY | GLUTEN-FREE | VEGAN

SERVES 4 This is a really simple soup, but with all the ginger the flavor is fantastic. You can jazz it up with garnishes like fresh lime juice. Ginger is also effective at soothing acid reflux, so this is a good soup to make if you're experiencing indigestion.

1. In a large pot over medium-high heat, heat the olive oil until it shimmers.

2. Add the ginger. Cook for about 1 minute, stirring until fragrant.

3. Stir in the broth, carrots, and salt. Bring to a boil. Reduce the heat to medium-low. Simmer for about 15 minutes, until the carrots are soft.

4. Carefully transfer the soup to a blender or food processor (or use an immersion blender). Blend until smooth. See the Tip for safe handling of hot soup when puréeing.

5. Garnish with the cilantro leaves.

Prep: 10 minutes
Cook: 18 minutes

2 tablespoons extra-virgin olive oil

2 tablespoons peeled, minced fresh ginger

7 cups Low-FODMAP Vegetable Broth (page 150)

10 carrots, chopped

½ teaspoon sea salt

2 tablespoons fresh cilantro leaves

COOKING TIP When puréeing hot liquids like soups, it is important to keep steam from building up in the container, or it can burst out and cause burns. (My mom did this once puréeing lentil soup—it ended up all over the kitchen. Fortunately, most of it missed my mom.) To safely purée the soup, plan to do it in batches. Do not fill the blender too full, and leave the top knob off the blender cap to let steam vent (or leave the oil chute out of the food processor). Fold a kitchen towel over four times, place it over the hole, and hold your hand over the towel to keep it in place. The folded towel will protect your hand. Then, start on low speed and slowly increase the speed to high. Stop blending and move the towel to allow steam to escape. Do this about three times while you purée the soup.

Per Serving (2 cups) Calories: 136; Total Fat: 7g; Saturated Fat: 1g; Carbohydrates: 18g; Fiber: 4g; Sodium: 347mg; Protein: 2g

Chicken Noodle Soup

30-MINUTE | GLUTEN-FREE

Prep: 10 minutes
Cook: 15 minutes

2 tablespoons Garlic Oil (page 153)

6 scallions, green parts only, chopped

3 carrots, chopped

1 red bell pepper, chopped

6 cups Low-FODMAP Poultry Broth (page 152)

½ teaspoon sea salt

⅛ teaspoon freshly ground black pepper

4 ounces gluten-free spaghetti, cooked according to instructions on package

4 cups chopped cooked chicken

SERVES 4 Using precooked rotisserie chicken makes this soup quick and easy for a busy weeknight meal. I often buy rotisserie chicken and shred the meat into 1-cup servings that I store in my freezer in zip-top bags. I can pull out just as much as I need for any given recipe, and give it a quick thaw in the microwave before using. To make this GERD friendly, see the Tip.

1. In a large pot over medium-high heat, heat the garlic oil until it shimmers.

2. Add the scallions, carrots, and bell pepper. Cook for 3 minutes, stirring occasionally.

3. Stir in the broth, salt, and pepper. Bring to a boil.

4. Add the spaghetti. Cook for 8 to 10 minutes, stirring occasionally, until the pasta is cooked. Drain.

5. Stir in the chicken. Cook for 2 minutes more.

SUBSTITUTION TIP To make this GERD friendly, replace the garlic oil with 1 tablespoon olive oil. Omit the black pepper, scallions, and the bell pepper. Replace the vegetables with 1 zucchini, chopped.

Per Serving (about 2½ cups) Calories: 441; Total Fat: 35g; Saturated Fat: 3g; Carbohydrates: 24g; Fiber: 2g; Sodium: 560mg; Protein: 52g

Turkey-Ginger Soup

30-MINUTE | GLUTEN-FREE

SERVES 4 This soup works well as a "refrigerator soup" base, where you dump in any low-FODMAP veggies you have sitting around. I typically make soups like this every few weeks to use up any extra veggies I have. Feel free to expand beyond what's listed in the recipe as long as the veggies you use are low-FODMAP. You can use the Monash University Low-FODMAP Diet app (see Resources, page 170) to determine what works and what doesn't. To make this GERD friendly, see the Tip.

Prep: 10 minutes
Cook: 17 minutes

2 tablespoons Garlic Oil (page 153)

1 pound ground turkey

6 scallions, green parts only, chopped

2 carrots, chopped

2 tablespoons peeled, minced fresh ginger

7 cups Low-FODMAP Poultry Broth (page 152)

½ teaspoon sea salt

⅛ teaspoon freshly ground black pepper

2 cups cooked brown rice

1. In a large pot over medium-high heat, heat the garlic oil until it shimmers.

2. Add the turkey. Cook for about 5 minutes, crumbling it with the back of a spoon, until browned.

3. Add the scallions, carrots, and ginger. Cook for 3 minutes, stirring.

4. Stir in the broth, salt, and pepper. Bring to a simmer. Cook for about 7 minutes, until the carrots soften.

5. Stir in the brown rice and cook for 2 minutes more to heat through.

SUBSTITUTION TIP To make this GERD friendly, replace the garlic oil with 1 tablespoon olive oil. Use only white meat ground turkey. Omit the black pepper.

Per Serving (about 3 cups) Calories: 482; Total Fat: 16g; Saturated Fat: 3g; Carbohydrates: 44g; Fiber: 3g; Sodium: 610mg; Protein: 44g

Vegetable Beef Soup

30-MINUTE | GLUTEN-FREE | LOW-CARB

Prep: 10 minutes
Cook: 15 minutes

1 pound ground beef

7 cups Low-FODMAP Poultry Broth (page 152)

6 scallions, green parts only, chopped

2 carrots, chopped

1 zucchini, chopped

1 red bell pepper, chopped

1 teaspoon dried thyme

½ teaspoon sea salt

⅛ teaspoon freshly ground black pepper

1 cup shredded cabbage

SERVES 4 When I was a kid, my mom would pop open a can of vegetable beef soup and serve it for lunch. I hated it. However, when she'd make a soup with the same vegetables and ground beef, I loved it. Kids. This is a riff on that soup from when I was a kid—the kind with the hamburger, minus the can. To make this GERD friendly, see the Tip.

1. In a large pot over medium-high heat, cook the ground beef for about 5 minutes, breaking it up with the back of a spoon, until browned.

2. Add the broth, scallions, carrots, zucchini, bell pepper, thyme, salt, and pepper. Bring the soup to a simmer and reduce the heat to medium. Cook for about 7 minutes, stirring occasionally, until the veggies are crisp-tender.

3. Stir in the cabbage. Cook for 3 minutes more.

SUBSTITUTION TIP To make this GERD friendly, use extra-lean (7 percent) ground beef. Replace the red bell pepper with an additional chopped zucchini. Omit the black pepper and reduce the serving size by half.

Per Serving (about 3 cups) Calories: 279; Total Fat: 7g; Saturated Fat: 3g; Carbohydrates: 11g; Fiber: 3g; Sodium: 465mg; Protein: 40g

Potato Leek Soup

5-INGREDIENT | 30-MINUTE | GLUTEN-FREE | VEGAN

SERVES 4 This is another easy-to-make soup. If you'd like to make it heartier with some animal protein, add some chopped bacon or ham. Otherwise, it's delicious as it is and really simple to prepare. The biggest issue may be cleaning the leeks (remember, green parts only—the whites are high in FODMAPs). See the Tip to ensure you remove all the dirt that's trapped in the leeks' layers.

Prep: 10 minutes
Cook: 13 minutes

6 cups Low-FODMAP Vegetable Broth (page 150)

5 russet potatoes, peeled and chopped

2 leeks, green parts only, thoroughly washed (see Tip) and chopped

½ teaspoon sea salt

⅛ teaspoon freshly ground black pepper

1. In a large pot over medium-high heat, stir together the broth, potatoes, leeks, salt, and pepper. Bring the soup to a boil. Reduce the heat to medium and simmer the soup for about 10 minutes, until the potatoes and leeks are soft.

2. In a blender or food processor, purée the soup, in batches if needed, until smooth. For safe puréeing of hot soup, see the Tip for Carrot and Ginger Soup, page 61.

SUBSTITUTION TIP To make this GERD friendly, omit the black pepper.

INGREDIENT TIP To clean the leek greens, thinly slice them and place them in a bowl of water. Agitate the water with your hands and allow it to settle. You'll notice dirt settling on the bottom of the bowl. Gently remove the leeks from the water, pour out the used water, and fill the bowl with clean water. Repeat the process until no more dirt settles to the bottom of the bowl. Pat the leeks dry with a paper towel.

Per Serving (about 2 cups) Calories: 234; Total Fat: <1g; Saturated Fat: 0g; Carbohydrates: 55g; Fiber: 7g; Sodium: 304mg; Protein: 5g

Lentil *and* Potato Soup

5-INGREDIENT | 30-MINUTE | GLUTEN-FREE | VEGAN

Prep: 10 minutes
Cook: 13 minutes

6 cups Low-FODMAP
Vegetable Broth (page 150)

4 Yukon Gold potatoes,
chopped

2 cups canned lentils, drained

1 carrot, chopped

1 teaspoon dried thyme

½ teaspoon sea salt

⅛ teaspoon freshly ground
black pepper

SERVES 4 Using canned lentils makes this soup ready in a snap. To minimize FODMAP load, Monash University recommends limiting lentils to a ½-cup serving, so keep that in mind with this soup. Each serving of the soup has about ½ cup of lentils, so save leftovers for another day. To make this IBS-D and GERD friendly, see the Tip.

1. In a large pot over medium-high heat, combine the broth, potatoes, lentils, carrot, thyme, salt, and pepper. Bring to a boil.

2. Reduce the heat to medium and simmer for about 10 minutes, until the potatoes are soft.

SUBSTITUTION TIP For IBS-D, reduce the lentils to 1 cup. Purée the soup to change the texture and help make it easier to digest. To make this GERD friendly, omit the black pepper and reduce the serving size by half.

Per Serving (about 3 cups) Calories: 497; Total Fat: 1g; Saturated Fat: 0g; Carbohydrates: 97g; Fiber: 32g; Sodium: 313mg; Protein: 5g

Greens *and* Lemon Soup

5-INGREDIENT | 30-MINUTE | GLUTEN-FREE | LOW-CARB | VEGAN

SERVES 4 Lemon adds a nice acidity to this tasty soup. If you don't like Swiss chard, use spinach or kale—or a combination of greens depending on what's available at your local market. This soup is high in antioxidants and other nutrients as well as flavor. To make this IBS-D friendly, see the Tip.

1. In a large pot over medium-high heat, heat the garlic oil until it shimmers.

2. Add the scallions and chard. Cook for 3 minutes, stirring.

3. Stir in the broth, salt, and pepper. Simmer for 10 minutes, stirring occasionally.

4. Squeeze in the lemon juice.

SUBSTITUTION TIP For IBS-D, replace the garlic oil with 2 tablespoons olive oil and omit the black pepper. Purée the soup to help make it easier to digest.

Per Serving (about 2 cups) Calories: 106; Total Fat: 7g; Saturated Fat: 1g; Carbohydrates: 11g; Fiber: 1g; Sodium: 387mg; Protein: 2g

Prep: 10 minutes
Cook: 15 minutes

2 tablespoons Garlic Oil (page 153)

5 scallions, green parts only, chopped

5 cups stemmed, chopped Swiss chard

6 cups Low-FODMAP Vegetable Broth (page 150)

½ teaspoon sea salt

¼ teaspoon freshly ground black pepper

Juice of 2 lemons

Smoked Gouda *and* Tomato Sandwich

5-INGREDIENT | 30-MINUTE | GLUTEN-FREE | VEGETARIAN

Prep: 5 minutes
Cook: 6 minutes

2 tablespoons garlic oil

4 slices gluten-free
sandwich bread

⅔ cup grated smoked
gouda cheese, divided

1 tomato, cut into
6 slices

SERVES 2 The grilled cheese is a simple sandwich, but it always makes a satisfying meal. Monash University lists about one-half cup of grated cheese as a safe amount to keep FODMAPs low so carefully measure the cheese and avoid eating any more cheese the same day to keep your FODMAP load within reasonable limits. If you have IBS-C, avoid this recipe.

1. Heat a non-stick skillet over medium-high heat.

2. Brush the outside of each bread slice with the garlic oil.

3. Place 2 pieces of bread, oil-side down, in the skillet. Top each with ⅓ cup cheese and three tomato slices. Top with the remaining 2 bread slices, oil side up.

4. Cook for about 3 minutes per side until the cheese melts and the bread browns on each side.

INGREDIENT TIP Grating the cheese helps it melt more evenly, and the smaller the shreds are, the better, so use your grater's smallest holes for grating the cheese.

Per Serving (1 sandwich) Calories: 536; Total Fat: 37g; Saturated Fat: 18g; Carbohydrates: 41g; Fiber: 9g; Sodium: 761mg; Protein: 15g

Egg Salad Sandwich

5-INGREDIENT | 30-MINUTE | GLUTEN-FREE | VEGETARIAN

SERVES 2 Egg salad is the perfect sandwich to take for meals on the go. To keep the bread from getting soggy (because nobody likes soggy bread), store the egg salad separately from the bread until you're ready to make the sandwich. Save time by purchasing hardboiled eggs at the grocery store. To make this Big 8 Allergen and GERD friendly, see the Tip.

1. In a small bowl, mix the eggs, scallions, mustard, mayonnaise, and salt.

2. Divide the egg salad between 2 bread slices and spread it out. Top with the remaining bread slices to make 2 sandwiches.

SUBSTITUTION TIP If you are allergic to eggs, replace them with ½ cup chopped tofu and increase the mustard to 2 teaspoons. To make this GERD friendly, omit the mayonnaise and use ¼ cup lactose-free plain yogurt instead.

Per Serving (1 sandwich) Calories: 532; Total Fat: 31g; Saturated Fat: 6g; Carbohydrates: 47g; Fiber: 9g; Sodium: 654mg; Protein: 19g

Prep: 5 minutes
Cook: 0 minutes

6 hardboiled eggs, peeled and chopped

3 scallions, green parts only, finely chopped

1 teaspoon Dijon mustard

¼ cup Low-FODMAP Mayonnaise (page 151)

¼ teaspoon sea salt

4 slices gluten-free sandwich bread

Pesto Ham Sandwich

5-INGREDIENT | 30-MINUTE | GLUTEN-FREE

Prep: 10 minutes
Cook: 0 minutes

4 slices gluten-free sandwich bread, toasted

4 tablespoons Macadamia Spinach Pesto (page 159), divided

4 ounces thinly sliced prosciutto, divided

4 pieces jarred roasted red pepper

SERVES 2 I love the combination of pesto and ham—there's just something so essentially Italian about the flavors. Here, I suggest using prosciutto, which makes this sandwich seem extra special, but you can use any type of ham, excepting honey-glazed or other sweetened varieties. If you do use honey-glazed ham, carefully trim away the outside edges where the honey is. To make this IBS-C and GERD friendly, see the Tip.

1. Spread 2 bread slices with 2 tablespoons pesto each.

2. Top each with half the prosciutto and half the roasted red pepper.

3. Top with the remaining bread slices.

SUBSTITUTION TIP If you have IBS-C, make the Macadamia Spinach Pesto (page 159) without cheese, or avoid this recipe. To make this sandwich GERD friendly, reduce the pesto to 2 tablespoons and replace the roasted red peppers with 2 tablespoons Olive Tapenade (page 164).

Per Serving (1 sandwich) Calories: 238; Total Fat: 12g; Saturated Fat: 2g; Carbohydrates: 25g; Fiber: 5g; Sodium: 790mg; Protein: 9g

Open-Faced Bacon, Tomato, and Cheese Sandwich

5-INGREDIENT | 30-MINUTE | GLUTEN-FREE

SERVES 2 When I was young, my mom used to make these sandwiches for me, and they were my absolute favorite. It's still one of my most beloved sandwiches today. There's just something about the flavor of bacon and tomato together—it's like they were made to go together. To save time, purchase precooked bacon. To make this IBS-C friendly, see the Tip.

Prep: 10 minutes
Cook: 6 minutes

6 bacon slices

2 slices gluten-free sandwich bread, toasted

1 tablespoon Garlic Oil (page 153)

1 tomato, sliced

½ cup grated Cheddar cheese, divided

1. In a large nonstick skillet over medium-high heat, cook the bacon for about 6 minutes, until crisp on both sides. Transfer to paper towels to drain.

2. Preheat the broiler to high and adjust a rack to the top position.

3. Brush one side of the toasted bread slices with garlic oil. Place the bread on a baking sheet, oiled-side up, and top with the tomato slices.

4. Top each sandwich with 3 bacon slices and sprinkle each with ¼ cup cheese.

5. Broil for about 3 minutes, until the cheese melts.

INGREDIENT TIP This sandwich is at its best when tomatoes are in season. Whenever possible, make it with freshly picked heirloom tomatoes from your garden or a local farmers' market.

SUBSTITUTION TIP If you have IBS-C, make this sandwich without the cheese, or avoid this recipe.

Per Serving (1 sandwich) Calories: 634; Total Fat: 48g; Saturated Fat: 19g; Carbohydrates: 22g; Fiber: 4g; Sodium: 1,516mg; Protein: 31g

Philly Steak Sandwich

30-MINUTE | GLUTEN-FREE

Prep: 10 minutes
Cook: 15 minutes

2 tablespoons Garlic Oil
(page 153)

1 green bell pepper, sliced

1 red bell pepper, sliced

6 scallions, green parts only,
sliced

6 ounces thinly sliced deli
roast beef, chopped

2 slices gluten-free sandwich
bread, toasted

½ cup grated Monterey Jack
cheese

SERVES 2 This open-faced knife-and-fork sandwich takes the flavors you love from classic Philly cheesesteak sandwiches and remakes them to be lower in FODMAPs so you can enjoy this classic American favorite without the stomach discomfort. To make this Big 8 Allergen and IBS-C friendly, see the Tip.

1. In a large nonstick skillet over medium-high heat, heat the garlic oil until it shimmers.

2. Add the green and red bell peppers and the scallions. Cook for about 7 minutes, stirring occasionally, until soft.

3. Add the roast beef, and cook for about 3 minutes more, until the beef is warmed through.

4. Preheat the broiler to high and adjust a rack to the top position.

5. Place the toasted bread on a baking sheet and top each with half the bell peppers and beef.

6. Sprinkle each with ¼ cup grated cheese.

7. Broil for about 3 minutes, until the cheese melts.

SUBSTITUTION TIP If you're allergic or intolerant to dairy or have IBS-C, omit the cheese and skip the broiling.

Per Serving (1 sandwich) Calories: 501; Total Fat: 31g; Saturated Fat: 9g; Carbohydrates: 30g; Fiber: 7g; Sodium: 641mg; Protein: 28g

Turkey-Tapenade Sandwich

30-MINUTE | GLUTEN-FREE

SERVES 2 In New Orleans, there's a popular sandwich called a muffaletta. It is a heavenly combination of meats, peppers, cheese, and olive tapenade stuffed into a large round loaf of bread. This is an easy FODMAP-friendly version that borrows some of the best flavors of the traditional muffaletta without all the work. To make this IBS-C and GERD friendly, see the Tip.

1. Spread 1 teaspoon mustard on each of 2 bread slices.

2. Top each with 2 pieces roasted red pepper, 2 tablespoons tapenade, 3 ounces turkey, 1 slice cheese, and the second bread slice.

SUBSTITUTION TIP If you have IBS-C, omit the cheese. To make this GERD friendly, omit the roasted red peppers.

Per Serving (1 sandwich) Calories: 487; Total Fat: 22g; Saturated Fat: 6g; Carbohydrates: 55g; Fiber: 10g; Sodium: 2,043mg; Protein: 22g

Prep: 10 minutes
Cook: 0 minutes

2 teaspoons Dijon mustard, divided

4 slices gluten-free sandwich bread, toasted

4 pieces jarred roasted red pepper

4 tablespoons Olive Tapenade (page 164), divided

6 ounces sliced deli turkey

2 slices Havarti cheese

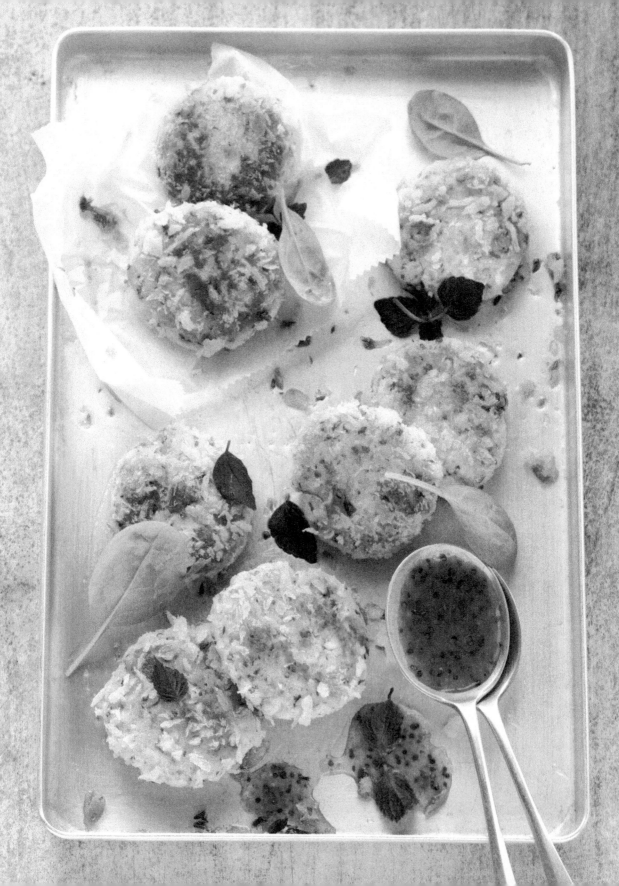

Vegetarian *and* Vegan Entrées

← *Tofu Burger Patties, page 84*

Stuffed Zucchini Boats

5-INGREDIENT | GLUTEN-FREE | VEGETARIAN

Prep: 10 minutes
Cook: 40 minutes

4 medium zucchini, halved lengthwise with the middles scooped out, chopped, and reserved

2 cups cooked brown rice

½ cup canned crushed tomatoes, drained

½ cup grated Parmesan cheese

¼ cup chopped fresh basil leaves

½ teaspoon sea salt

⅛ teaspoon freshly ground black pepper

SERVES 4 This doesn't require much work time—only 5 to 10 minutes, but it does take a while in the oven. The result is a fragrant, flavorful vegetarian main dish. If you're vegan or have IBS-C, leave out the cheese. To make this GERD friendly, see the Tip.

1. Preheat the oven to 400°F.

2. Place the zucchini halves on a rimmed baking sheet, cut-side up.

3. In a medium bowl, stir together the brown rice, reserved chopped zucchini, tomatoes, Parmesan cheese, basil, salt, and pepper. Spoon the mixture into the zucchini boats.

4. Bake for 40 to 45 minutes, until the zucchini are soft.

SUBSTITUTION TIP To make this GERD friendly, replace the crushed tomatoes with ¼ cup chopped black olives and ¼ cup low-FODMAP Vegetable Broth (page 150).

Per Serving (2 pieces) Calories: 262; Total Fat: 5g; Saturated Fat: 2g; Carbohydrates: 46g; Fiber: 5g; Sodium: 447mg; Protein: 11g

Spanish Rice

30-MINUTE | GLUTEN-FREE | VEGAN

SERVES 4 Using precooked brown rice makes this recipe come together quickly, and it's packed with delicious flavors. This makes a tasty main dish or a versatile side dish. To make this GERD friendly, see the Tip.

1. In a large skillet over medium-high heat, heat the garlic oil until it shimmers.

2. Add the scallions. Cook for 3 minutes, stirring occasionally.

3. Stir in the brown rice, tomatoes, broth, olives, pine nuts, oregano, salt, and pepper. Cook for about 5 minutes more, stirring, until warmed through.

SUBSTITUTION TIP To make this GERD friendly, replace the tomatoes with an additional ½ cup Low-FODMAP Vegetable Broth (page 150). Replace the garlic oil with 1 tablespoon olive oil. Omit the black pepper.

Per Serving (1½ cups) Calories: 399; Total Fat: 22g; Saturated Fat: 2g; Carbohydrates: 46g; Fiber: 6g; Sodium: 506mg; Protein: 8g

Prep: 10 minutes
Cook: 10 minutes

2 tablespoons Garlic Oil (page 153)

6 scallions, green parts only, chopped

2 cups hot cooked brown rice

1 cup canned crushed tomatoes, drained

½ cup Low-FODMAP Vegetable Broth (page 150)

½ cup chopped black olives

½ cup pine nuts

1 teaspoon dried oregano

½ teaspoon sea salt

¼ teaspoon freshly ground black pepper

Vegetable Stir-Fry

5-INGREDIENT | 30-MINUTE | GLUTEN-FREE | LOW-CARB | VEGAN

Prep: 10 minutes
Cook: 10 minutes

2 tablespoons Garlic Oil
(page 153)

2⅔ cups chopped firm tofu

8 scallions, green parts only,
chopped

2 cups broccoli florets

½ cup Stir-Fry Sauce
(page 161)

SERVES 4 Tofu won't increase your FODMAP load, provided you stick to a serving of about ⅔ cup of chopped *firm* tofu per day. Don't use silken tofu here, which is high in oligosaccharides. Serve over plain brown rice or Spanish Rice (page 77), if desired. To make this GERD friendly, see the Tip.

1. In a large skillet over medium-high heat, heat the garlic oil until it shimmers.

2. Add the tofu, scallions, and broccoli. Cook for about 7 minutes, stirring frequently, until the broccoli is crisp-tender.

3. Stir in the stir-fry sauce. Cook for about 3 minutes, stirring, until it thickens.

SUBSTITUTION TIP To make this GERD friendly, omit the garlic oil and instead use 1 tablespoon olive oil. Omit the scallions, and follow the GERD friendly variation for Stir-Fry Sauce (page 161).

Per Serving (2 cups) Calories: 231; Total Fat: 14g; Saturated Fat: 3g; Carbohydrates: 14g; Fiber: 4g; Sodium: 426mg; Protein: 16g

Peanut Butter Soba Noodles

30-MINUTE | GLUTEN-FREE | VEGAN

SERVES 4 Soba noodles are made from buckwheat flour. Don't let the name give you pause—buckwheat is not related to wheat. It is gluten-free and low in FODMAPs. Read labels to ensure the soba noodles you use are made with 100 percent buckwheat flour and don't include wheat as an ingredient. To make this Big 8 Allergen friendly, see the Tip. If you have GERD, avoid this.

1. In a small bowl (or a blender), whisk together the peanut butter, soy sauce, lime juice, garlic oil, ginger, and stevia until smooth.

2. In a large serving bowl, combine the hot noodles and sauce and toss to coat.

SUBSTITUTION TIP If you are allergic to peanuts, substitute an equal amount of almond butter.

Per Serving (about 2 cups) Calories: 357; Total Fat: 13g; Saturated Fat: 3g; Carbohydrates: 49g; Fiber: 2g; Sodium: 1,501mg; Protein: 17g

Prep: 15 minutes
Cook: 0 minutes

6 tablespoons sugar-free natural peanut butter

¼ cup low-sodium gluten-free soy sauce

2 tablespoons freshly squeezed lime juice

1 tablespoon Garlic Oil (page 153)

1 teaspoon peeled and grated fresh ginger

1 packet stevia

8 ounces soba noodles, cooked according to the package directions, drained, and hot

Potato Frittata

GLUTEN-FREE | LOW-CARB | VEGETARIAN

Prep: 10 minutes
Cook: 35 minutes

6 eggs, beaten

2 tablespoons unsweetened almond milk

½ teaspoon sea salt

⅛ teaspoon freshly ground black pepper

2 tablespoons Garlic Oil (page 153)

2 russet potatoes, sliced

½ cup grated Parmesan cheese

4 cherry tomatoes, quartered

Arugula, for garnishing (optional)

SERVES 2 Frittatas are a great way to add veggies to your meals, so add any low-FODMAP veggies (see list on page 12 or consult the Monash University Low-FODMAP Diet app) that sound tasty. This version uses nutritious fresh baby spinach for a healthy dose of antioxidants. To make this IBS-C and GERD friendly, see the Tip.

1. Preheat the broiler to high.

2. In a medium bowl, whisk together the eggs, almond milk, salt, and pepper. Set it aside.

3. In a large (12-inch) ovenproof skillet heat over medium-high heat, heat the garlic oil until it shimmers.

4. Add the potatoes. Cook for about 20 minutes, stirring occasionally, until soft.

5. Carefully pour the egg mixture over the potatoes. Cook for about 5 minutes, until the eggs start to set around the edges. With a heat-proof spatula, pull the edges away from the pan and tilt the pan to allow the egg mixture to flow into any spaces you've made. Cook for about 5 minutes more, until the edges set again. Sprinkle with the cheese and top with the tomatoes.

6. Place the skillet under the broiler for 3 to 5 minutes, until the frittata sets and puffs and the cheese melts.

7. Garnish with arugula (if using).

SUBSTITUTION TIP If you have IBS-C, omit the cheese. To make this GERD friendly, replace the garlic oil with 1 tablespoon olive oil. Use 3 whole eggs and 6 egg whites in place of the 6 whole eggs for the frittata, and reduce the Parmesan cheese to ¼ cup.

Per Serving (½ frittata) Calories: 445; Total Fat: 37g; Saturated Fat: 13g; Carbohydrates: 5g; Fiber: 1g; Sodium: 954mg; Protein: 27g

Crustless Spinach Quiche

5-INGREDIENT | **30-MINUTE** | **GLUTEN-FREE** | **LOW-CARB** | **VEGETARIAN**

Prep: 5 minutes
Cook: 20 minutes

Nonstick cooking spray

6 eggs, beaten

¼ cup unsweetened almond milk

½ teaspoon sea salt

⅛ teaspoon freshly ground black pepper

1 teaspoon dried thyme

2 cups (2 [8-ounce] boxes) frozen spinach, thawed and squeezed of excess moisture

½ cup grated Swiss cheese

SERVES 4 It doesn't take long to mix up this quiche because it doesn't require a crust. With about 5 minutes of prep time and 20 minutes in the oven, you'll have a fragrant, flavorful meal in less than 30 minutes. It also freezes well, so it's a good make-ahead dish for busy weeks. To make this IBS-C and GERD friendly, see the Tip.

1. Preheat the oven to 350°F.

2. Spray a 9-inch pie pan with nonstick cooking spray.

3. In a medium bowl, whisk together the eggs, almond milk, salt, pepper, and thyme.

4. Fold in the spinach and cheese. Pour the mixture into the prepared pie pan.

5. Bake for 20 to 25 minutes, until the quiche sets.

SUBSTITUTION TIP If you have IBS-C, omit the cheese. To make this GERD friendly, omit the black pepper. Use 3 whole eggs and 6 egg whites in place of the 6 whole eggs, and reduce the Swiss cheese to ¼ cup.

Per Serving (¼ quiche) Calories: 187; Total Fat: 14g; Saturated Fat: 8g; Carbohydrates: 3g; Fiber: <1g; Sodium: 368mg; Protein: 13g

Cheese Strata

5-INGREDIENT | GLUTEN-FREE | VEGETARIAN

SERVES 4 Strata is a casserole made with a mixture of eggs, soaked bread, and cheese. It's similar to a bread pudding, but savory instead of sweet. For the best results, prepare the bread mixture the night before and let it soak overnight in the refrigerator so the eggs really soak into the bread. In the morning, simply pop it into the oven. If you're pressed for time, bake it as is without the overnight soaking. To make this GERD friendly, see the Tip.

1. Preheat the oven to 350°F.

2. Spray a 9-by-5-inch loaf pan with nonstick cooking spray.

3. In a medium bowl, whisk together the eggs, almond milk, salt, and pepper.

4. Fold in the bread until it is coated with the egg mixture.

5. Fold in the cheese.

6. Pour the mixture into the prepared dish and bake for 30 to 35 minutes, until set.

SUBSTITUTION TIP To make this GERD friendly, omit the black pepper and reduce the cheese to ½ cup. If you have IBS-C, avoid this recipe.

Per Serving (¼ strata) Calories: 402; Total Fat: 29g; Saturated Fat: 18g; Carbohydrates: 28g; Fiber: 6g; Sodium: 628mg; Protein: 12g

Prep: 10 minutes
Cook: 30 minutes

Nonstick cooking spray

3 eggs, beaten

1 cup unsweetened almond milk

½ teaspoon sea salt

⅛ teaspoon freshly ground black pepper

5 slices gluten-free sandwich bread, crusts removed, cut into cubes

¾ cup grated Monterey Jack cheese

Tofu Burger Patties

30-MINUTE | GLUTEN-FREE | VEGETARIAN

Prep: 15 minutes
Cook: 10 minutes

8 ounces firm tofu,
mashed with a fork

4 scallions, green parts only,
minced

1 cup rolled oats

1 egg, beaten

2 teaspoons ground cumin

2 teaspoons chili powder

½ teaspoon sea salt

¼ teaspoon freshly ground
black pepper

Nonstick cooking spray

SERVES 4 Firm tofu and veggies make a great patty
that you can enjoy on a salad or in a gluten-free
bun for burger night. This fast recipe packs a good
wallop of flavor. Serve with a simple side salad for
a complete meal. To make this GERD friendly, see
the Tip.

1. In a medium bowl, stir together the tofu, scallions, oats, egg,
cumin, chili powder, salt, and pepper. Form the mixture into
4 patties.

2. Spray a large nonstick skillet with cooking spray and place
it over medium-high heat.

3. Add the patties and cook for about 5 minutes per side,
until browned on both sides.

SUBSTITUTION TIP To make this GERD friendly, omit the
chili powder, scallions, and pepper. Along with the cumin,
add ¼ cup chopped fresh cilantro leaves and 1 teaspoon
ground ginger.

Per Serving (1 patty) Calories: 146; Total Fat: 5g; Saturated Fat: 1g;
Carbohydrates: 17g; Fiber: 4g; Sodium: 275mg; Protein: 10g

Pasta *with* Pesto Sauce

5-INGREDIENT | 30-MINUTE | GLUTEN-FREE | VEGETARIAN

SERVES 4 Pasta with pesto is a delicious, quick, and easy choice when those are your requirements for mealtime. A fun alternative for this dish (and a lower-carb version, too) is to make noodles from zucchini with a spiralizer, but any gluten-free pasta will work here. To make this IBS-C friendly, see the Tip. If you have GERD, avoid this recipe.

1. In the warm pot that you used to cook the pasta, toss the noodles with the pesto.

2. Sprinkle with the cheese.

Prep: 15 minutes
Cook: 0 minutes

8 ounces gluten-free angel hair pasta, cooked according to the package instructions. Drained.

1 recipe Macadamia Spinach Pesto (page 159)

¼ cup grated Parmesan cheese

COOKING TIP To make zucchini noodles for this dish: Spiralize 4 zucchini or cut them into ribbons with a vegetable peeler. Sauté the noodles in 2 tablespoons Garlic Oil (page 153) over medium-high heat for about 5 minutes before tossing with the pesto.

SUBSTITUTION TIP If you have IBS-C, omit the cheese in this dish and make the Macadamia Spinach Pesto (page 159) without cheese, or avoid this recipe.

Per Serving (2 ounces pasta with ¼ cup pesto) Calories: 449; Total Fat: 25g; Saturated Fat: 6g; Carbohydrates: 46g; Fiber: 3g; Sodium: 444mg; Protein: 13g

Pasta *with* Tomato *and* Lentil Sauce

30-MINUTE | GLUTEN-FREE | VEGAN

Prep: 5 minutes
Cook: 10 minutes

2 tablespoons Garlic Oil
(page 153)

6 scallions, green parts only, chopped

2 cups canned lentils, drained

1½ cups canned crushed tomatoes, undrained

1 tablespoon dried Italian seasoning

½ teaspoon sea salt

Pinch red pepper flakes

¼ cup chopped fresh basil leaves

8 ounces gluten-free pasta (any shape), cooked according to the package directions, drained

SERVES 4 Lentils add protein and texture to this tasty tomato sauce. When tossed with pasta, it makes a hearty meal. Remember, to minimize FODMAP load, limit your lentil consumption to ½ cup per day and use only canned lentils.

1. In a large skillet over medium-high heat, heat the garlic oil until it shimmers.

2. Add the scallions and cook for 3 minutes.

3. Stir in the lentils, tomatoes, Italian seasoning, salt, and red pepper flakes. Simmer for 5 minutes, stirring.

4. Stir in the basil.

5. Add the hot pasta and toss to coat.

INGREDIENT TIP If you don't have dried Italian seasoning, substitute 1 teaspoon dried thyme, 1 teaspoon dried oregano, and 1 teaspoon dried basil.

Per Serving (2 ounces pasta with ½ cup sauce) Calories: 426; Total Fat: 3g; Saturated Fat: 0g; Carbohydrates: 73g; Fiber: 34g; Sodium: 461mg; Protein: 28g

Tofu *and* Red Bell Pepper Quinoa

5-INGREDIENT | GLUTEN-FREE | VEGAN

SERVES 4 This one-pot meal is packed with vegetarian protein from both the quinoa and the tofu. With red bell peppers, it's also a full meal—protein, grain, and veggie all in one. To make this GERD friendly, see the Tip.

Prep: 5 minutes
Cook: 21 minutes
Rest: 5 minutes

2 tablespoons Garlic Oil (page 153)

1 red bell pepper, chopped

6 ounces firm tofu, chopped

1 cup quinoa, rinsed well

2 cups Low-FODMAP Vegetable Broth (page 150)

1 teaspoon dried thyme

½ teaspoon sea salt

¼ teaspoon freshly ground black pepper

1. In a large saucepan over medium-high heat, heat the garlic oil until it shimmers.

2. Add the bell pepper and the tofu. Cook for about 5 minutes, stirring, until the pepper is soft.

3. Add the quinoa. Cook for 1 minute, stirring.

4. Add the broth, thyme, salt, and pepper. Bring to a boil. Reduce the heat to medium and simmer for 15 minutes.

5. Turn off the heat. Cover the pot and let it sit for 5 minutes more.

6. Fluff with a fork.

SUBSTITUTION TIP To make this GERD friendly, replace the garlic oil with 1 tablespoon olive oil. Replace the red bell pepper with 2 chopped carrots. Omit the black pepper.

Per Serving (about 2 cups) Calories: 276; Total Fat: 12g; Saturated Fat: 2g; Carbohydrates: 31g; Fiber: 4g; Sodium: 624mg; Protein: 12g

Eggplant *and* Chickpea Curry

30-MINUTE | GLUTEN-FREE | VEGAN

Prep: 10 minutes
Cook: 15 minutes

2 tablespoons Garlic Oil
(page 153)

6 scallions, green parts only,
minced

2 cups chopped eggplant

1 cup canned chickpeas,
drained

1 cup unsweetened
almond milk

1 tablespoon curry powder

¼ teaspoon freshly ground
black pepper

SERVES 4 This simple curry can be eaten alone or spooned over steamed brown rice. Eggplant, at about ½ cup per serving, won't raise your FODMAP load above a safe level, and canned chickpeas are safe at about ¼ cup. So, because of the amounts of each in this recipe, save leftovers for another day to maintain a reasonable FODMAP load. To make this GERD friendly, see the Tip.

1. In a large skillet over medium-high heat, heat the garlic oil until it shimmers.

2. Add the scallions and eggplant. Cook for about 5 minutes, stirring, until the eggplant is soft.

3. Add the chickpeas, almond milk, curry powder, and pepper. Bring to a boil. Reduce the heat to medium-low and simmer for 10 minutes.

SUBSTITUTION TIP To make this GERD friendly, replace the garlic oil with 1 tablespoon olive oil and omit the black pepper.

Per Serving (about 2 cups) Calories: 275; Total Fat: 11g; Saturated Fat: 1g; Carbohydrates: 36g; Fiber: 12g; Sodium: 62mg; Protein: 11g

Tempeh Lettuce Wraps

30-MINUTE | GLUTEN-FREE | VEGAN

SERVES 4 This great family-style meal starts with sautéed, spiced tempeh and ends with raw garnishes to add crunch and flavor. Everyone can fill their own lettuce wraps with whatever sounds good. To make this GERD friendly, see the Tip.

1. In a large skillet over medium-high heat, heat the garlic oil until it shimmers.

2. Add the tempeh and five-spice powder. Cook for 3 to 4 minutes, stirring, until the tempeh is warmed through.

3. In a small bowl, whisk the peanut butter, broth, soy sauce, and ginger. Stir the sauce into the tempeh. Cook for 3 minutes more, stirring.

4. Serve with the lettuce leaves to wrap and the garnishes (if using) on the side.

SUBSTITUTION TIP To make this GERD friendly, replace the garlic oil with 1 tablespoon olive oil. Replace the Chinese five-spice powder with 2 teaspoons ground star anise.

Per Serving (about 1 cup filling plus 2 lettuce leaves, without garnishes)
Calories: 433; Total Fat: 27g; Saturated Fat: 6g; Carbohydrates: 21g; Fiber: 2g;
Sodium: 367mg; Protein: 36g

Prep: 10 minutes
Cook: 8 minutes

2 tablespoons Garlic Oil (page 153)

4 cups chopped tempeh

1 tablespoon Chinese five-spice powder

¼ cup creamy sugar-free natural peanut butter

¼ cup Low-FODMAP Vegetable Broth (page 150)

1 tablespoon gluten-free soy sauce

1 teaspoon ground ginger

8 large lettuce leaves

Minced scallions, green parts only, for garnishing (optional)

Chopped fresh cilantro leaves, for garnishing (optional)

Bean sprouts, for garnishing (optional)

Chopped peanuts, for garnishing (optional)

Pineapple Fried Rice

30-MINUTE | GLUTEN-FREE | VEGAN

Prep: 5 minutes
Cook: 10 minutes

2 tablespoons Garlic Oil
(page 153)

6 scallions, green parts only,
finely chopped

½ cup canned water
chestnuts, drained

1 tablespoon peeled and
grated fresh ginger

3 cups cooked brown rice

2 cups canned pineapple
(in juice), drained, ¼ cup
juice reserved

2 tablespoons gluten-free
soy sauce

¼ cup chopped fresh
cilantro leaves

SERVES 4 Precooked brown rice and canned pineapple pair here for a tropical-tasting and easy recipe. It makes a delicious dinner served hot, or pack it and eat it cold for lunch. Simple!

1. In a large skillet over medium-high heat, heat the garlic oil until it shimmers.

2. Add the scallions, water chestnuts, and ginger. Cook for 5 minutes, stirring.

3. Add the brown rice, pineapple, reserved pineapple juice, and soy sauce. Cook for 5 minutes, stirring, until the rice is warmed through.

4. Stir in the cilantro.

INGREDIENT TIP Use fresh pineapple here if you prefer. If you do, replace the pineapple juice with ¼ cup freshly squeezed lime juice.

Per Serving (about 2 cups) Calories: 413; Total Fat: 9g; Saturated Fat: 1g; Carbohydrates: 77g; Fiber: 4g; Sodium: 396mg; Protein: 7g

Zucchini Pizza Bites

5-INGREDIENT | 30-MINUTE | GLUTEN-FREE | LOW-CARB | VEGETARIAN

SERVES 4 Who needs pizza crust when you can make mini pizzas from zucchini slices? This recipe gives you the flavors of pizza but without the crust, so it's a tasty, low-carb, low-FODMAP, vegetarian meal or snack. Add your favorite toppings to this basic cheese pizza recipe. To make this IBS-C friendly, see the Tip.

Prep: 10 minutes
Cook: 15 minutes

2 medium zucchini, cut into ¼-inch-thick slices

1 cup tomato sauce

2 tablespoons Garlic Oil (page 153)

2 teaspoons dried Italian seasoning

½ teaspoon sea salt

1 cup grated mozzarella cheese

1. Preheat the oven to 350°F.

2. Line two rimmed baking sheets with parchment paper. Arrange the zucchini slices in a single layer on the prepared sheets.

3. In a small bowl, whisk the tomato sauce, garlic oil, Italian seasoning, and salt. Spread the sauce on the zucchini slices.

4. Top with the cheese.

5. Bake for about 15 minutes, until the zucchini is soft and the cheese melts.

COOKING TIP You can make larger pizza bites using eggplant slices. If you do, stick to one slice of eggplant per serving (about ½ cup chopped eggplant) to keep the FODMAP load low.

SUBSTITUTION TIP If you have IBS-C, omit the cheese.

Per Serving (about 8 pieces) Calories: 124; Total Fat: 6g; Saturated Fat: 3g; Carbohydrates: 9g; Fiber: 2g; Sodium: 736mg; Protein: 10g

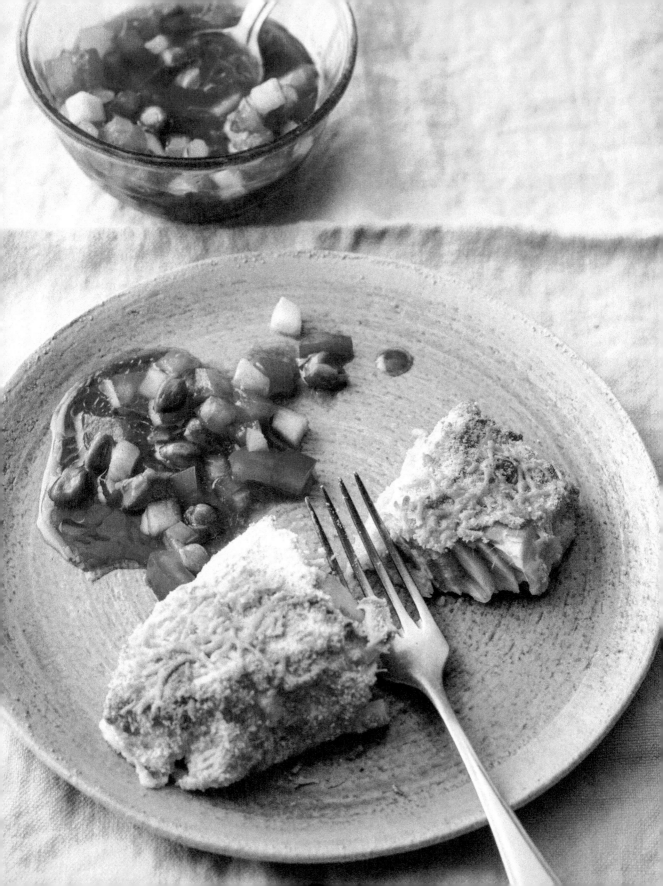

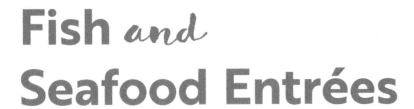

Fish *and* Seafood Entrées

← *Breaded Fish Fillets with Spicy Pepper Relish, page 102*

Sautéed Shrimp *with* Cilantro-Lime Rice

5-INGREDIENT | 30-MINUTE | GLUTEN-FREE

Prep: 10 minutes
Cook: 10 minutes

3 tablespoons Garlic Oil
(page 153)

1 pound medium shrimp,
peeled and deveined

2 cups cooked brown rice

¼ cup Cilantro-Lime
Vinaigrette (page 154)

½ teaspoon sea salt

SERVES 4 Although this has a little lime juice in it, if you suffer from acid reflux, the small amount of vinaigrette used here likely will not aggravate your condition. If you are especially sensitive to citrus juice, have plain rice with cilantro stirred in instead. To make this GERD friendly, see the Tip.

1. In a large nonstick skillet over medium-high heat, heat the garlic oil until it shimmers.

2. Add the shrimp. Cook for about 5 minutes, stirring occasionally, until the shrimp is pink.

3. Stir in the rice, vinaigrette, and salt. Cook for 2 minutes more, stirring.

SUBSTITUTION TIP To make this GERD friendly, replace the garlic oil with 2 tablespoons olive oil.

Per Serving (4 ounces shrimp with ¼ cup rice) Calories: 360; Total Fat: 11g; Saturated Fat: 2g; Carbohydrates: 38g; Fiber: 2g; Sodium: 494mg; Protein: 28g

Chili-Lime Shrimp *and* Bell Peppers

30-MINUTE | GLUTEN-FREE

SERVES 4 Sweet shrimp gets a little heat with chili powder and cayenne pepper in this low-carb main course. If you prefer things on the milder side, adjust the heat by reducing or omitting the cayenne—or pump it up if you like a bit of fire with your shrimp. With cayenne, a little goes a long way, so add extra cautiously. To make this Big 8 Allergen friendly, see the Tip.

1. In a large nonstick skillet over medium-high heat, heat the garlic oil until it shimmers.

2. Add the bell pepper. Cook for 3 minutes, stirring.

3. Add the shrimp. Cook for about 5 minutes, stirring occasionally, until it is pink.

4. Stir in the lime juice, chili powder, salt, cayenne, and pepper. Cook for 2 minutes.

SUBSTITUTION TIP If you are allergic to shellfish, replace the shrimp with cod and cook it for about 5 minutes. You can also use chopped chicken breast, cooking the chicken for about 7 minutes.

Per Serving (4 ounces shrimp with ¼ cup bell pepper) Calories: 360; Total Fat: 11g; Saturated Fat: 2g; Carbohydrates: 38g; Fiber: 2g; Sodium: 494mg; Protein: 28g

Prep: 10 minutes
Cook: 10 minutes

3 tablespoons Garlic Oil (page 153)

1 red bell pepper, chopped

1 pound shrimp, peeled and deveined

Juice of 1 lime

1 teaspoon chili powder

½ teaspoon sea salt

⅛ teaspoon cayenne pepper

⅛ teaspoon freshly ground black pepper

Lemon-Pepper Shrimp

5-INGREDIENT | 30-MINUTE | GLUTEN-FREE | LOW-CARB

Prep: 5 minutes
Cook: 8 minutes

2 tablespoons Garlic Oil
(page 153)

1 pound medium shrimp,
shelled and deveined

Juice of 2 lemons

½ teaspoon sea salt

½ teaspoon freshly ground
black pepper

SERVES 4 This shrimp is delicious as a main dish, tossed with pasta, or as a topping for a simple salad with any of the vinaigrettes in chapter 9 (see page 149). Save prep time by purchasing already shelled and deveined shrimp in the freezer section of your grocery store. To make this Big 8 Allergen friendly, see the Tip.

1. In a large nonstick skillet over medium-high heat, heat the garlic oil until it shimmers.

2. Add the shrimp. Cook for about 5 minutes, stirring occasionally, until it is pink.

3. Squeeze in the lemon juice, then add the salt and pepper. Simmer for 3 minutes more.

SUBSTITUTION TIP If you are allergic to shellfish, replace the shrimp with 1 pound white fish, such as cod or halibut, cut into 1-inch pieces.

Per Serving (about 4 ounces) Calories: 119; Total Fat: 2g; Saturated Fat: 0g; Carbohydrates: 2g; Fiber: 0g; Sodium: 494mg; Protein: 25g

Pan-Seared Scallops *with* Sautéed Kale

5-INGREDIENT | 30-MINUTE | GLUTEN-FREE | LOW-CARB

SERVES 4 Serving these scallops on a nest of citrus-scented kale makes a flavorful meal. Scallops cook very quickly—about three minutes per side to keep them from getting tough. Set them aside tented with aluminum foil to keep warm, as your kale cooks in the same pan. To make this GERD friendly, see the Tip.

Prep: 10 minutes
Cook: 15 minutes

2 tablespoons extra-virgin olive oil

1 pound sea scallops

½ teaspoon sea salt

⅛ teaspoon freshly ground black pepper

3 cups stemmed, chopped kale leaves

Juice of 1 orange

Zest of 1 orange

1. In a large nonstick skillet over medium-high heat, heat the olive oil until it shimmers. Swirl the pan to coat it with the oil.

2. Season the scallops with salt and pepper. Add them to the hot skillet and cook for about 3 minutes per side. Transfer the scallops to a platter and tent with foil to keep warm. Return the skillet to the heat.

3. Add the kale to the skillet. Cook for about 5 minutes, stirring.

4. Add the orange juice and zest. Cook for 3 minutes more.

5. Serve the scallops on top of the sautéed kale.

SUBSTITUTION TIP To make this GERD friendly, replace the orange juice with ½ cup Low-FODMAP Vegetable Broth (page 150) but keep the orange zest.

INGREDIENT TIP To prepare the scallops, remove the tough tendon along the side of each with a sharp paring knife. Otherwise, it will shrink and toughen while cooking.

Per Serving (about 4 scallops and ½ cup kale) Calories: 199; Total Fat: 8g; Saturated Fat: 1g; Carbohydrates: 11g; Fiber: <1g; Sodium: 439mg; Protein: 21g

Snapper *with* Tropical Salsa

30-MINUTE | GLUTEN-FREE | LOW-CARB

Prep: 15 minutes
Cook: 8 minutes

2 tablespoons extra-virgin olive oil

1 pound snapper, quartered

1 teaspoon sea salt, divided

⅛ teaspoon freshly ground black pepper

1 papaya, chopped

1 cup chopped pineapple

1 jalapeño pepper, seeded and minced

1 tablespoon chopped fresh cilantro leaves

Juice of 1 lime

SERVES 4 Tropical fruit makes a fantastic salsa to accompany fish. This simple snapper dish is a delicious summer main course, and it goes well with rice or quinoa and a side salad for a light and very flavorful low-FODMAP meal. To make this Big 8 Allergen friendly, see the Tip.

1. In a large nonstick skillet over medium-high heat, heat the olive oil until it shimmers.

2. Season the snapper with ½ teaspoon salt and the pepper. Add it to the skillet and cook for about 4 minutes per side, until the fish is opaque.

3. In a medium bowl, gently stir together the papaya, pineapple, jalapeño, cilantro, lime juice, and remaining ½ teaspoon salt.

4. Serve the salsa on top of the snapper.

SUBSTITUTION TIP If you are allergic to fish, season 1 pound sea scallops with salt and pepper. Cook in the hot olive oil for about 3 minutes per side and serve with the salsa.

Per Serving (4 ounces snapper with about ½ cup salsa) Calories: 236; Total Fat: 8g; Saturated Fat: 1g; Carbohydrates: 14g; Fiber: 2g; Sodium: 565mg; Protein: 27g

Herb-Crusted Halibut

5-INGREDIENT | 30-MINUTE | GLUTEN-FREE | LOW-CARB

SERVES 4 Here in the Pacific Northwest, fresh Alaskan halibut is plentiful, but I understand it may not be so easy to find in other parts of the country. If needed, replace the halibut with your favorite white fish that is readily available where you live. To make this GERD friendly, see the Tip.

1. Preheat the oven to 450°F.

2. Place the halibut fillets on a nonstick rimmed baking sheet.

3. In a small bowl, whisk the parsley with the mustard, garlic oil, thyme, salt, and pepper. Spread the mustard mixture over the halibut.

4. Bake the halibut for about 15 minutes, until opaque.

SUBSTITUTION TIP To make this GERD friendly, replace the garlic oil with 1 tablespoon olive oil and omit the black pepper.

Per Serving (4 ounces) Calories: 189; Total Fat: 8g; Saturated Fat: 1g; Carbohydrates: 1g; Fiber: <1g; Sodium: 416mg; Protein: 27g

Prep: 10 minutes
Cook: 15 minutes

1 pound halibut, quartered

½ cup finely chopped fresh parsley leaves

2 tablespoons Dijon mustard

2 tablespoons Garlic Oil (page 153)

2 teaspoons dried thyme

½ teaspoon sea salt

⅛ teaspoon freshly ground black pepper

Lemon-Dill Cod *on a* Bed of Spinach

5-INGREDIENT | 30-MINUTE | GLUTEN-FREE | LOW-CARB

Prep: 10 minutes
Cook: 15 minutes

3 tablespoons Garlic Oil
(page 153)

1 pound cod, quartered

½ teaspoon sea salt

⅛ teaspoon freshly ground
black pepper

Juice of 1 lemon

2 tablespoons chopped
fresh dill

3 cups fresh baby spinach

SERVES 4 Cod is an affordable and readily available fish found in most grocery stores. If there's something fresh and local that looks better to you, feel free to substitute any other white-fleshed fish. To make this GERD friendly, see the Tip.

1. In a large nonstick skillet over medium-high heat, heat the garlic oil until it shimmers.

2. Season the cod with salt and pepper. Add it to the skillet and cook for about 4 minutes per side, until opaque.

3. Sprinkle on the lemon juice and dill. Cook for 2 minutes more, spooning the sauce over the fish. With tongs, transfer the fish to a plate and tent with aluminum foil to keep warm. Return the skillet to the heat.

4. Add the spinach to the pan. Cook for about 3 minutes, stirring occasionally, until wilted.

5. Serve the cod on top of the spinach.

SUBSTITUTION TIP To make this GERD friendly, replace the lemon juice with ¼ cup Low-FODMAP Vegetable Broth (page 150) and add the grated zest of 1 lemon. Omit the black pepper. Replace the garlic oil with 2 tablespoons olive oil.

Per Serving (4 ounces plus ½ cup spinach) Calories: 222; Total Fat: 12g; Saturated Fat: 2g; Carbohydrates: 2g; Fiber: <1g; Sodium: 347mg; Protein: 27g

Sesame-Crusted Cod

30-MINUTE | GLUTEN-FREE | LOW-CARB

SERVES 4 Sesame seeds, up to about 5 tablespoons per day, won't tip your FODMAP load, so they make a great crust for simple cod fillets. Ginger and Chinese hot mustard powder (the prepared mustard contains wheat flour, but the powder doesn't) give this dish a classic Asian-inspired flavor profile. To make this GERD friendly, see the Tip.

1. Preheat the oven to 400°F.

2. In a small bowl, whisk together the eggs, garlic oil, ginger, sesame oil, and Chinese hot mustard powder.

3. In another small bowl, mix the sesame seeds, salt, and pepper.

4. Dip the cod into the egg mixture and into the seasoned sesame seeds to coat. Place it on a rimmed baking sheet. Bake for 15 minutes, until opaque.

SUBSTITUTION TIP To make this GERD friendly, omit the garlic oil, hot mustard powder, and black pepper, and replace the garlic oil with ½ tablespoon olive oil.

Per Serving (4 ounces) Calories: 274; Total Fat: 13g; Saturated Fat: 2g; Carbohydrates: 6g; Fiber: 2g; Sodium: 356mg; Protein: 32g

Prep: 10 minutes
Cook: 15 minutes

2 eggs, beaten

1 tablespoon Garlic Oil (page 153)

1 tablespoon peeled and grated fresh ginger

1 teaspoon sesame oil

½ teaspoon Chinese hot mustard powder

½ cup sesame seeds

½ teaspoon sea salt

⅛ teaspoon freshly ground black pepper

1 pound cod, quartered

Breaded Fish Fillets
with Spicy Pepper Relish

30-MINUTE | GLUTEN-FREE | LOW-CARB

Prep: 10 minutes
Cook: 15 minutes

2 cups gluten-free bread crumbs (see Tip)

1¼ teaspoons sea salt, divided

1 teaspoon dried thyme

⅛ teaspoon freshly ground black pepper

2 eggs, beaten

1 tablespoon Dijon mustard

1 pound cod, cut into 8 pieces

1 red bell pepper, chopped

2 tablespoons capers, drained and rinsed

1 jalapeño pepper, minced

Juice of 1 lime

¼ teaspoon red pepper flakes

SERVES 4 If it's fish and chips you crave, this version is easy to make—you can have it on the table in 30 minutes. Combine it with Parmesan Potato Wedges (page 139) for a classic pub-style dinner. To make this GERD friendly, see the Tip.

1. Preheat the oven to 425°F.

2. In a small bowl, whisk the bread crumbs, 1 teaspoon salt, thyme, and pepper.

3. In another small bowl, whisk the eggs and mustard.

4. Dip the fish into the egg mixture and into the breading mixture to coat. Place the fish on a nonstick rimmed baking sheet. Bake for about 15 minutes, until the crust is golden and the fish is opaque.

5. While the fish cooks, in a small bowl, stir together the bell pepper, capers, jalapeño, lime juice, red pepper flakes, and the remaining ¼ teaspoon salt.

6. Serve the fish topped with the relish.

SUBSTITUTION TIP To make this GERD friendly, omit the black pepper and the relish.

INGREDIENT TIP Purchase gluten-free bread crumbs or make your own in a blender or food processor by pulsing stale gluten-free sandwich bread (crusts removed) until roughly chopped.

Per Serving (2 pieces with about 2 tablespoons relish) Calories: 209; Total Fat: 3g; Saturated Fat: <1g; Carbohydrates: 13g; Fiber: 2g; Sodium: 699mg; Protein: 30g

Tuna Lemon Pasta

30-MINUTE | GLUTEN-FREE

Prep: 10 minutes
Cook: 10 minutes

2 tablespoons Garlic Oil
(page 153)

6 scallions, green parts only,
chopped

1 red bell pepper, chopped

8 ounces water-packed tuna,
drained and flaked

Juice of 1 lemon

½ teaspoon sea salt

8 ounces gluten-free pasta,
cooked according to
the package directions
and drained

SERVES 4 This pasta is not only quick, but it's also budget friendly—think of it as a lighter tuna casserole. With just a few ingredients, you get a colorful and tasty dish that's sure to become a favorite of tuna fans everywhere. Choose water-packed tuna, or substitute 8 ounces of your favorite cooked fish or shellfish. To make this GERD friendly, see the Tip.

1. In a large nonstick skillet over medium-high heat, heat the garlic oil until it shimmers.

2. Add the scallions and bell pepper. Cook for 5 minutes, stirring.

3. Stir in the tuna, lemon juice, and salt. Cook for 3 minutes more, stirring.

4. Toss with the hot pasta.

SUBSTITUTION TIP To make this GERD friendly, replace the lemon juice with ¼ cup Low-FODMAP Vegetable Broth (page 150) and add the grated zest of 1 lemon. In place of the garlic oil, use 1 tablespoon olive oil.

Per Serving (about 2 cups) Calories: 349; Total Fat: 13g; Saturated Fat: 2g; Carbohydrates: 35g; Fiber: 1g; Sodium: 284mg; Protein: 22g

Tuna *and* Pineapple Burgers

30-MINUTE | GLUTEN-FREE

SERVES 4 Just because it's burger night doesn't mean you need to have the same old hamburger. Shake things up with this tuna and pineapple burger. It's an interesting twist on typical burger night fare, and the sweetness of the pineapple is delicious with the tuna. To make this Big 8 Allergen friendly, see the Tip.

Prep: 15 minutes
Cook: 10 minutes

1 pound canned tuna, flaked

½ cup gluten-free bread crumbs

1 egg, beaten

¼ cup plus 2 tablespoons Low-FODMAP Mayonnaise (page 151), divided

Zest of 1 lemon

½ teaspoon sea salt

⅛ teaspoon freshly ground black pepper

2 tablespoons Garlic Oil (page 153)

3 tablespoons Teriyaki Sauce (page 163)

4 canned pineapple slices, packed in water, drained

4 gluten-free hamburger buns

1. In a large bowl, mix the tuna, bread crumbs, egg, 2 tablespoons mayonnaise, lemon zest, salt, and pepper until thoroughly combined. Form the tuna mixture into 4 patties.

2. In a large nonstick skillet over medium-high heat, heat the garlic oil until it shimmers.

3. Add the patties and cook for 5 minutes per side.

4. While the burgers cook, in a small bowl, whisk together the teriyaki sauce and remaining ¼ cup mayonnaise. Spread the sauce on the buns.

5. Place 1 cooked burger in each bun and top with 1 pineapple slice.

SUBSTITUTION TIP If you are allergic to fish, replace the tuna with 1 pound chopped cooked shrimp.

Per Serving (1 burger with pineapple and 1 bun) Calories: 495; Total Fat: 18g; Saturated Fat: 4g; Carbohydrates: 42g; Fiber: 2g; Sodium: 1,270mg; Protein: 39g

Orange-Ginger Salmon

5-INGREDIENT | 30-MINUTE | GLUTEN-FREE | LOW-CARB

Prep: 5 minutes
Marinating: 10 minutes
Cook: 12 minutes

¼ cup Garlic Oil (page 153)

Juice of 2 oranges

2 tablespoons gluten-free soy sauce

1 tablespoon peeled and grated fresh ginger

1 pound salmon fillet, quartered

SERVES 4 Salmon is plentiful, affordable, and easy to make into a great oven-baked entrée with very little prep. Just marinate the salmon for about 10 minutes, pop it in the oven, and dinner will be ready in under 30 minutes. Serve with steamed vegetables or sautéed greens and precooked brown rice. To make this Big 8 Allergen friendly, see the Tip.

1. Preheat the oven to 450°F.

2. In a shallow baking dish, whisk together the garlic oil, orange juice, soy sauce, and ginger.

3. Place the salmon, flesh-side down, in the marinade. Marinate for 10 minutes.

4. Place the salmon, skin-side up, on a rimmed baking sheet. Bake for 12 to 15 minutes, until opaque.

SUBSTITUTION TIP If you are allergic to fish, substitute 1 pound large sea scallops. Marinate them for 5 minutes per side in the marinade. Reduce the oven temperature to 425°F and bake the scallops for about 10 minutes, until opaque.

Per Serving (about 4 ounces) Calories: 282; Total Fat: 20g; Saturated Fat: 3g; Carbohydrates: 5g; Fiber: 0g; Sodium: 553mg; Protein: 23g

Easy Salmon Cakes

5-INGREDIENT | 30-MINUTE | GLUTEN-FREE | LOW-CARB

SERVES 4 Canned salmon is incredibly high in nutrients and very flavorful. These salmon cakes are terrific by themselves, or atop a salad dressed with a vinaigrette, or served on gluten-free buns. You can also use smoked salmon in the recipe; if you do, eliminate the sea salt. To make this GERD friendly, see the Tip.

Prep: 10 minutes
Cook: 10 minutes

1 pound canned salmon, flaked

½ cup gluten-free bread crumbs

1 egg, beaten

1 tablespoon Dijon mustard

1 tablespoon chopped fresh dill

½ teaspoon sea salt

⅛ teaspoon freshly ground black pepper

1. Preheat the oven to 375°F.

2. Line a baking sheet with parchment paper and set it aside.

3. In a large bowl, mix the salmon and the bread crumbs.

4. In a small bowl, whisk together the egg, mustard, dill, salt, and pepper. Fold this into the salmon and bread crumbs. Form the salmon mixture into 4 patties and place them on the prepared sheet.

5. Bake for 5 minutes, flip, and bake for 5 minutes more, until the patties are golden.

SUBSTITUTION TIP To make this GERD friendly, omit the black pepper and reduce the mustard to 2 teaspoons.

Per Serving (1 patty) Calories: 184; Total Fat: 8g; Saturated Fat: 1g; Carbohydrates: 4g; Fiber: 0g; Sodium: 362mg; Protein: 24g

Creamy Smoked Salmon Pasta

30-MINUTE | GLUTEN-FREE

Prep: 10 minutes
Cook: 9 minutes

2 tablespoons Garlic Oil
(page 153)

6 scallions, green parts only,
chopped

2 tablespoons capers, drained

12 ounces smoked salmon,
flaked

¾ cup unsweetened
almond milk

2 tablespoons chopped
fresh dill

⅛ teaspoon freshly ground
black pepper

8 ounces gluten-free pasta,
cooked according to the
package directions
and drained

SERVES 4 Smoked salmon and capers are a classic combination, and this pasta capitalizes on that delicious flavor pairing. If capers are a bit too salty for you, rinse them well in a wire mesh sieve and pat them dry before adding them to the pasta. To make this GERD friendly, see the Tip.

1. In a large nonstick skillet over medium-high heat, heat the garlic oil until it shimmers.

2. Add the scallions and capers. Cook for 2 minutes, stirring.

3. Add the salmon and cook for 2 minutes more.

4. Stir in the almond milk, dill, and pepper. Simmer for 3 minutes.

5. Toss with the hot pasta.

SUBSTITUTION TIP To make this GERD friendly, omit the capers, black pepper, and garlic oil and replace it with 1 tablespoon olive oil.

Per Serving (about 2 cups) Calories: 287; Total Fat: 6g; Saturated Fat: 1g; Carbohydrates: 35g; Fiber: 1g; Sodium: 1,920mg; Protein: 23g

Teriyaki Salmon

5-INGREDIENT | 30-MINUTE | GERD FRIENDLY | GLUTEN-FREE | LOW-CARB

SERVES 4 Need a meal in a hurry that's still good for you? This salmon dish requires minimal prep but is full of flavor. Make the Teriyaki Sauce (page 163) ahead of time and you can keep it refrigerated for up to 2 weeks, or freeze it for up to 6 months. Serve this with rice and steamed veggies for a complete meal. To make this Big 8 Allergen friendly, see the Tip.

Prep: 5 minutes
Cook: 10 minutes

1 pound salmon, quartered

¼ cup Teriyaki Sauce (page 163)

1. Preheat the oven to 425°F.

2. Place the salmon on a nonstick rimmed baking sheet.

3. Brush the salmon with the sauce and bake for about 10 minutes, until opaque.

SUBSTITUTION TIP If you are allergic to fish, brush boneless, skinless chicken breasts with the teriyaki sauce. Bake them at 425°F for 20 to 30 minutes, or until cooked through.

Per Serving (4 ounces) Calories: 166; Total Fat: 7g; Saturated Fat: 1g; Carbohydrates: 3g; Fiber: 0g; Sodium: 740mg; Protein: 23g

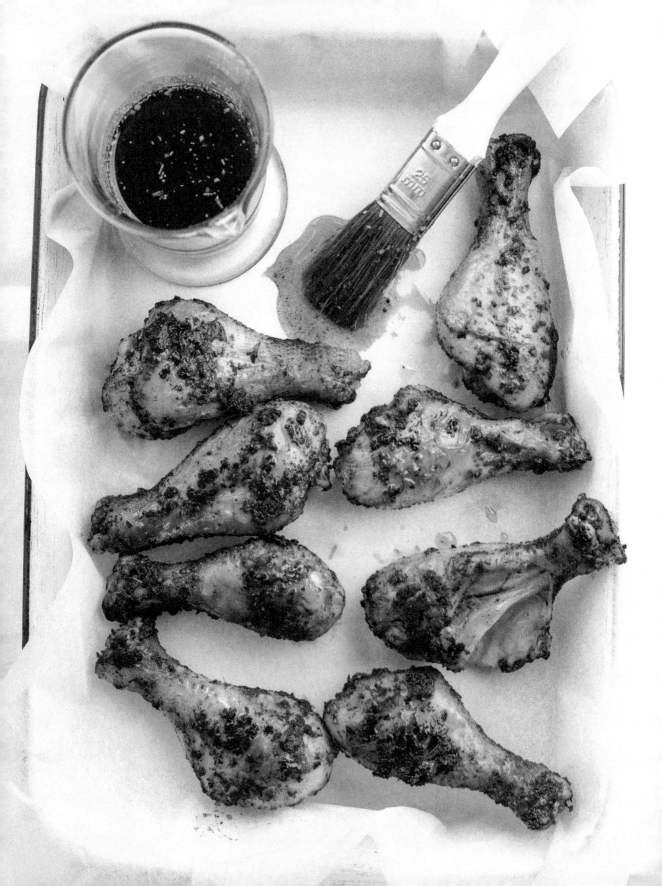

SEVEN

Poultry *and* Meat Entrées

← *Chimichurri Chicken Drumsticks, page 116*

Barbecue Chicken

5-INGREDIENT | GLUTEN-FREE | LOW-CARB

Prep: 5 minutes
Cook: 30 minutes

8 chicken drumsticks

1 recipe Homemade
Barbecue Sauce (page 160)

SERVES 4 Most traditional barbecue sauces and rubs are filled with ingredients people with IBS just can't eat. Using Homemade Barbecue Sauce (page 160), this recipe proves you don't need FODMAPs—or an outdoor grill—to make tasty barbecue chicken. While this recipe uses drumsticks, you can use any cut of chicken—just adjust the baking time accordingly (see Tip). Serve with Quick Creamy Coleslaw (page 49). Keep any leftovers in the refrigerator for up to 3 days.

1. Preheat the oven to 375°F.

2. Place the chicken pieces in a large baking dish and brush them on all sides with the barbecue sauce.

3. Bake for about 30 minutes, or until the juices run clear.

COOKING TIP Chicken thighs will take about the same amount of time to cook; add 5 to 10 minutes for boneless, skinless breasts.

Per Serving (2 drumsticks) Calories: 155; Total Fat: 6g; Saturated Fat: 1g; Carbohydrates: 5g; Fiber: 1g; Sodium: 328mg; Protein: 26g

Chicken *with* Macadamia Spinach Pesto

5-INGREDIENT | 30-MINUTE | GLUTEN-FREE | LOW-CARB

SERVES 4 One of the easiest ways to jazz up chicken is to serve it with an easy, flavorful sauce, such as this recipe using Macadamia Spinach Pesto (page 159). It's also full of antioxidants, and goes great with spiralized zucchini noodles. To make this IBS-C friendly, see the Tip.

Prep: 5 minutes
Cook: 10 minutes

4 (4- to 6-ounce) boneless, skinless chicken breast halves, pounded to ½-inch thickness (see Tip)

½ teaspoon sea salt

⅛ teaspoon freshly ground black pepper

2 tablespoons extra-virgin olive oil

½ cup Macadamia Spinach Pesto (page 159)

1. Season the chicken breast with salt and pepper.

2. In a large nonstick skillet over medium-high heat, heat the olive oil until it shimmers.

3. Add the chicken and cook for about 4 minutes per side, until the juices run clear.

4. Serve with the pesto spooned over the top.

COOKING TIP Put the chicken breasts between two pieces of parchment paper or plastic wrap before you pound them to keep the chicken from splattering.

SUBSTITUTION TIP If you have IBS-C, make the Macadamia Spinach Pesto (page 159) without cheese, or avoid this recipe.

Per Serving (½ chicken breast with 2 tablespoons pesto) Calories: 237; Total Fat: 22g; Saturated Fat: 4g; Carbohydrates: 2g; Fiber: <1g; Sodium: 443mg; Protein: 9g

Chicken *and* Rice *with* Peanut Sauce

30-MINUTE | GLUTEN-FREE

Prep: 10 minutes
Cook: 10 minutes

2 tablespoons Garlic Oil
(page 153)

1 pound boneless skinless
chicken thigh meat,
cut into strips

½ cup sugar-free natural
peanut butter

½ cup coconut milk

2 tablespoons gluten-free
soy sauce

1 tablespoon peeled and
grated fresh ginger

Juice of 1 lime

2 cups cooked brown rice

SERVES 4 Add low-FODMAP veggies of your choice (see the list on page 12) to this quick stir-fry if you'd like to make it a full meal, or serve with a side of steamed vegetables or a salad. You can also use boneless skinless chicken breast in place of the thigh meat if you prefer. To make this Big 8 Allergen and GERD friendly, see the Tip.

1. In a large nonstick skillet over medium-high heat, heat the garlic oil until it shimmers.

2. Add the chicken and cook for about 6 minutes, stirring occasionally, until browned.

3. In a small bowl, whisk the peanut butter, coconut milk, soy sauce, ginger, and lime juice. Add this to the chicken.

4. Mix in the rice. Cook for 3 minutes more, stirring.

SUBSTITUTION TIP If you are allergic to peanuts, replace the peanut butter with almond butter. To make this GERD friendly, replace the lime juice with 1 additional tablespoon soy sauce; replace the garlic oil with 1 tablespoon olive oil; replace the coconut milk with ½ cup light coconut milk.

Per Serving (4 ounces chicken, ½ cup rice, ¼ cup peanut sauce) Calories: 718; Total Fat: 40g; Saturated Fat: 13g; Carbohydrates: 46g; Fiber: 5g; Sodium: 757mg; Protein: 46g

Chicken Tenders

5-INGREDIENT | 30-MINUTE | GLUTEN-FREE

SERVES 4 Serve this comfort food classic with Parmesan Potato Wedges (page 139), as well as a salad or steamed veggies. If you prefer to dip your tenders, make some Homemade Barbecue Sauce (page 160) or Teriyaki Sauce (page 163), or whisk together some gluten-free soy sauce into low-FODMAP Mayonnaise (page 151) and dip away. To make this GERD friendly, see the Tip.

Prep: 10 minutes
Cook: 15 minutes

1 cup gluten-free bread crumbs

1 teaspoon dried thyme

½ teaspoon sea salt

⅛ teaspoon freshly ground black pepper

2 eggs, beaten

1 tablespoon Dijon mustard

1 pound boneless skinless chicken breast, cut into strips

1. Preheat the oven to 425°F.

2. In a medium bowl, mix the bread crumbs, thyme, salt, and pepper.

3. In a small bowl, whisk the eggs and mustard.

4. Dip the chicken strips into the egg mixture and into the bread crumb mixture to coat. Place them on a nonstick rimmed baking sheet.

5. Bake for 15 to 20 minutes, until the breading is golden and the juices run clear.

SUBSTITUTION TIP To make this GERD friendly, omit the black pepper and Dijon mustard.

Per Serving (4 ounces) Calories: 183; Total Fat: 5g; Saturated Fat: 2g; Carbohydrates: 20g; Fiber: 2g; Sodium: 526mg; Protein: 13g

Chimichurri Chicken Drumsticks

5-INGREDIENT | GLUTEN-FREE

Prep: 10 minutes
Marinating: 8 hours
Cook: 30 minutes

8 chicken drumsticks

1 cup Chimichurri Sauce
(page 158), divided

SERVES 4 These chicken drumsticks make delicious use of classic Argentinean-style Chimichurri Sauce (page 158). Just marinate the drumsticks in some chimichurri before cooking. Rice is a great accompaniment for this dish, along with additional chimichurri.

1. In a gallon-size zip-top bag, combine the drumsticks with ½ cup chimichurri sauce. Seal the bag and shake to coat. Refrigerate for 8 hours.

2. Preheat the oven to 375°F.

3. Line a rimmed baking sheet with parchment paper.

4. Remove the drumsticks from the bag, pat the marinade off with a paper towel (a little will be left, which is okay), and place them on the prepared baking sheet. Bake for about 30 minutes, or until the juices run clear.

5. Serve with the remaining ½ cup chimichurri sauce on the side.

INGREDIENT TIP Use chicken thighs for this dish if you prefer. Increase the cooking time to about 40 minutes.

Per Serving (2 drumsticks with about 2 tablespoons chimichurri)
Calories: 401; Total Fat: 11g; Saturated Fat: 3g; Carbohydrates: 39g; Fiber: 3g;
Sodium: 968mg; Protein: 35g

Rosemary-Lemon Chicken Thighs

5-INGREDIENT | GLUTEN-FREE | LOW-CARB

SERVES 4 Lemon and rosemary is a delicious and fragrant flavor combination. When it's used as a coating for roasted chicken thighs, it makes the skin uniquely crispy and caramelized. To make this GERD friendly, see the Tip.

Prep: 10 minutes
Cook: 30 minutes

8 chicken thighs

1 tablespoon chopped fresh rosemary leaves

1 teaspoon sea salt

Zest of 1 lemon

¼ teaspoon freshly ground black pepper

1. Preheat the oven to 375°F.

2. Line a rimmed baking sheet with parchment paper and place the chicken thighs, skin-side up, on the sheet.

3. In a small bowl, mix the rosemary, salt, lemon zest, and pepper. Sprinkle this over the thighs.

4. Bake for about 30 minutes, or until the juices run clear.

SUBSTITUTION TIP The lemon zest in this recipe is GERD friendly (lemon juice is not), but omit the black pepper to make it entirely GERD friendly.

Per Serving (2 thighs) Calories: 535; Total Fat: 21g; Saturated Fat: 6g; Carbohydrates: <1g; Fiber: 0g; Sodium: 709mg; Protein: 81g

Chicken Carbonara

30-MINUTE | GLUTEN-FREE

Prep: 15 minutes
Cook: 5 minutes

2 tablespoons Garlic Oil
(page 153)

8 ounces boneless skinless
chicken breast, chopped

3 bacon slices, chopped

8 ounces gluten-free pasta,
cooked according to
the package directions
and drained

3 eggs, beaten

2 tablespoons unsweetened
almond milk

½ teaspoon sea salt

⅛ teaspoon freshly ground
black pepper

½ cup grated Parmesan
cheese

SERVES 4 Carbonara is a Roman-style bacon-and-egg pasta, and one of my favorite quick pasta dishes. Sometimes, I add steamed broccoli or chopped zucchini so I have a full meal in a single serving of pasta. To make this meal IBS-C and GERD friendly, see the Tip.

1. In a large nonstick skillet over medium-high heat, heat the garlic oil until it shimmers.

2. Add the chicken and bacon. Cook for about 5 minutes, until the bacon is crisp and chicken is cooked through.

3. Add the cooked pasta to the pan, stir to combine, and turn off the heat.

4. In a small bowl, whisk the eggs, almond milk, salt, and pepper. Stir the egg mixture into the hot pasta. The hot ingredients and residual heat from the stove will cook the eggs and turn it into a sauce.

5. Toss with the cheese.

SUBSTITUTION TIP If you have IBS-C, omit the cheese. To make this GERD friendly, omit the black pepper and garlic oil (no need to replace it—it's just for flavor). Reduce the cheese to ¼ cup.

Per Serving (about 2 cups) Calories: 727; Total Fat: 32g; Saturated Fat: 12g; Carbohydrates: 33g; Fiber: 0g; Sodium: 1,105mg; Protein: 73g

Turkey Dijon

5-INGREDIENT | 30-MINUTE | GLUTEN-FREE | LOW-CARB

SERVES 4 Pounding the turkey into thin pieces makes this dish a breeze to prepare. A simple and quick pan sauce coats the turkey for added flavor. Serve with a side of Orange-Maple Glazed Carrots (page 53) and some cooked brown rice for a complete meal. To make this GERD friendly, see the Tip.

Prep: 10 minutes
Cook: 15 minutes

2 tablespoons Garlic Oil (page 153)

4 (4-ounce) turkey cutlets, pounded to ¼-inch thickness

2 tablespoons Dijon mustard

1 cup Low-FODMAP Poultry Broth (page 152)

1 tablespoon cornstarch

½ teaspoon sea salt

⅛ teaspoon freshly ground black pepper

1. In a large nonstick skillet over medium-high heat, heat the garlic oil until it shimmers.

2. Add the turkey and cook for about 4 minutes per side, until the juices run clear. Transfer the turkey to a plate and tent with aluminum foil to keep warm. Return the skillet to the heat.

3. In a small bowl, whisk the broth, cornstarch, salt, and pepper. Whisk this into the hot skillet and cook for 1 to 2 minutes, whisking until the sauce thickens.

4. Serve the turkey with the sauce spooned over the top.

SUBSTITUTION TIP To make this GERD friendly, omit the black pepper and garlic oil and replace with 2 tablespoons olive oil.

Per Serving (1 cutlet) Calories: 270; Total Fat: 13g; Saturated Fat: 3g; Carbohydrates: 3g; Fiber: 0g; Sodium: 420mg; Protein: 34g

Sweet-*and*-Sour Turkey Meatballs

30-MINUTE | GLUTEN-FREE

Prep: 10 minutes
Cook: 12 minutes

1 pound ground turkey

½ cup gluten-free
bread crumbs

¼ cup chopped fresh
cilantro leaves

1 egg, beaten

2 tablespoons peeled and
grated fresh ginger

1 teaspoon sea salt

½ teaspoon freshly ground
black pepper

2 tablespoons Garlic Oil
(page 153)

1 recipe Sweet-and-Sour
Sauce (page 162)

SERVES 4 These meatballs are a fast, simple, and low-FODMAP way to enjoy the flavor of Chinese-style sweet-and-sour sauce. Serve with cooked brown rice and stir-fried low-FODMAP veggies (see the list on page 12). To make this GERD friendly, see the Tip.

1. In a large bowl, mix the turkey, bread crumbs, cilantro, egg, ginger, salt, and pepper. Form the turkey mixture into about 16 (1-inch) meatballs.

2. In a large nonstick skillet over medium-high heat, heat the garlic oil until it shimmers.

3. Add the meatballs and cook, turning, for about 8 minutes, or until the juices run clear and the meatballs are browned.

4. Stir in the sweet-and-sour sauce. Cook for 2 minutes more, stirring to coat the meatballs in the sauce.

COOKING TIP To keep the meat from sticking to your hands as you roll the meatballs, wet them with cold water, rewetting as you work.

SUBSTITUTION TIP To make this GERD friendly, omit the black pepper and garlic oil and replace with 2 tablespoons olive oil.

Per Serving (4 ounces, about 4 meatballs) Calories: 396; Total Fat: 15g; Saturated Fat: 3g; Carbohydrates: 32g; Fiber: 2g; Sodium: 1,041mg; Protein: 36g

Turkey *and* Red Pepper Burgers

5-INGREDIENT | 30-MINUTE | GLUTEN-FREE

SERVES 4 Turkey burgers can often be a bit bland—but not these. The red pepper mayonnaise, which adds a sweet piquancy, contributes lots of flavor to this great option for burger night. Make it a complete meal by serving with Parmesan Potato Wedges (page 139) and a salad. To make this GERD friendly, see the Tip.

Prep: 10 minutes
Cook: 10 minutes

1 pound ground turkey

½ teaspoon sea salt

⅛ teaspoon freshly ground black pepper

2 tablespoons extra-virgin olive oil

¼ cup Low-FODMAP Mayonnaise (page 151)

2 jarred roasted red peppers, minced

4 gluten-free hamburger buns

1. Form the turkey into 4 patties and season them with salt and pepper.

2. In a large nonstick skillet over medium-high heat, heat the olive oil until it shimmers.

3. Add the burgers and cook for about 5 minutes per side, until browned.

4. In a small bowl, whisk the mayonnaise and red peppers. Spread the mixture on the buns and add the cooked patties.

SUBSTITUTION TIP To make this GERD friendly, omit the roasted red peppers and instead stir in 2 tablespoons Olive Tapenade (page 164). Omit the mayonnaise.

Per Serving (1 burger with mayonnaise and bun) Calories: 468; Total Fat: 26g; Saturated Fat: 4g; Carbohydrates: 27g; Fiber: 1g; Sodium: 753mg; Protein: 36g

Mexican-Style Ground Beef *and* Rice

30-MINUTE | GLUTEN-FREE

Prep: 10 minutes
Cook: 15 minutes

2 tablespoons Garlic Oil
(page 153)

1 pound 85 percent lean
ground beef (see Tip)

6 scallions, green parts only,
chopped

½ cup water

1 tablespoon chili powder

1 teaspoon dried cumin

½ teaspoon sea salt

⅛ teaspoon freshly ground
black pepper

2 cups cooked brown rice

¼ cup chopped fresh
cilantro leaves

SERVES 4 If you like tacos, you'll enjoy this chili-spiced ground beef mixed with brown rice. It's a tasty meal that also freezes and travels well. Make a batch ahead of time and take with you when you need a meal on the go.

1. In a large nonstick skillet over medium-high heat, heat the garlic oil until it shimmers.

2. Add the ground beef and scallions. Cook for about 6 minutes, crumbling the beef with the back of a spoon, until it is browned.

3. Stir in the water, chili powder, cumin, salt, and pepper. Cook for 2 minutes more, stirring, until the spices are mixed in.

4. Stir in the brown rice and cilantro. Cook for 2 minutes more to heat.

INGREDIENT TIP Don't choose the leanest ground beef here—you'll want some fat to blend with the spices. Try 85 percent lean, which is also a great ratio for burgers.

Per Serving (about 2 cups) Calories: 458; Total Fat: 16g; Saturated Fat: 4g; Carbohydrates: 39g; Fiber: 3g; Sodium: 335mg; Protein: 39g

Spaghetti *and* Meat Sauce

30-MINUTE | GLUTEN-FREE

SERVES 4 Spaghetti is one of my favorite go-to meals. It's also uncannily easy to make a rich sauce for it quickly, particularly with ground beef, herbs, and spices. Serve with a side salad.

1. In a large nonstick skillet over medium-high heat, heat the garlic oil until it shimmers.

2. Add the ground beef and cook for about 6 minutes, crumbling it with the back of a spoon, until browned.

3. Stir in the tomato sauce and oregano.

4. In a small bowl, whisk together the broth, cornstarch, salt, and red pepper flakes. Add this to the skillet and cook for about 2 minutes, stirring, until the sauce begins to thicken.

5. Stir in the basil.

6. Toss with the hot spaghetti.

INGREDIENT TIP Substitute hot Italian sausage for a spicier sauce.

Per Serving (about 1 cup spaghetti with ½ cup sauce) Calories: 468; Total Fat: 16g; Saturated Fat: 4g; Carbohydrates: 37g; Fiber: 1g; Sodium: 835mg; Protein: 43g

Prep: 15 minutes
Cook: 10 minutes

2 tablespoons Garlic Oil (page 153)

1 pound ground beef

1 cup tomato sauce

1 teaspoon dried oregano

1 cup Low-FODMAP Poultry Broth (page 152)

1 tablespoon cornstarch

½ teaspoon sea salt

Pinch red pepper flakes

¼ cup chopped fresh basil leaves

8 ounces gluten-free spaghetti, cooked according to the package directions and drained

Quick Meatloaf Patties

30-MINUTE | GLUTEN-FREE | LOW-CARB

Prep: 10 minutes
Cook: 10 minutes

1 pound ground beef

½ cup gluten-free
bread crumbs

1 egg, beaten

1 tablespoon Dijon mustard

1 tablespoon Worcestershire
sauce

1 teaspoon dried thyme

1 teaspoon sea salt

⅛ teaspoon freshly ground
black pepper

2 tablespoons extra-virgin
olive oil

SERVES 4 Meatloaf takes a long time to cook in the oven—about an hour or longer, which is great when you have the time. By making patties and cooking them in a skillet, you get the same flavors, but in much less time. Serve with Mashed Potatoes (page 54) for a classic meal.

1. In a large bowl, combine the ground beef, bread crumbs, egg, mustard, Worcestershire sauce, thyme, salt, and pepper. Mix well. Form the meat mixture into 4 patties.

2. In a large nonstick skillet over medium-high heat, heat the olive oil until it shimmers.

3. Add the patties and cook for about 5 minutes per side, until browned on both sides.

INGREDIENT TIP To ensure the ground beef mixes well with the flavorings, mix with clean hands instead of a spoon.

Per Serving (1 patty) Calories: 295; Total Fat: 15g; Saturated Fat: 4g; Carbohydrates: 2g; Fiber: 0g; Sodium: 644mg; Protein: 36g

20-Minute Pulled Pork

5-INGREDIENT | 30-MINUTE | GLUTEN-FREE | LOW-CARB

SERVES 4 If you make the Homemade Barbecue Sauce (page 160) ahead of time, you can make this pulled pork with little preparation. Using a cut-up pork tenderloin instead of the traditional slow-cooked whole pork shoulder is what makes this recipe fast and easy. Serve with Quick Creamy Coleslaw (page 49) and gluten-free hamburger buns for a low-FODMAP version of an American classic.

Prep: 5 minutes
Cook: 20 minutes

1 recipe Homemade Barbecue Sauce (page 160)

1 pound pork tenderloin, cut into 5 pieces

1. In a large pot over medium-high heat, heat the barbecue sauce until it simmers.

2. Add the pork and cook for 20 minutes.

3. With two forks, carefully shred the pork and mix it with the barbecue sauce.

INGREDIENT TIP You can also use ground pork for this recipe. Brown it in a skillet, add the barbecue sauce, and bring it to a simmer, which will take about 5 minutes.

Per Serving (4 ounces) Calories: 244; Total Fat: 11g; Saturated Fat: 2; Carbohydrates: 4g; Fiber: 1g; Sodium: 318mg; Protein: 31g

Quick Steak Tacos

30-MINUTE | GLUTEN-FREE

Prep: 15 minutes
Cook: 15 minutes

2 tablespoons Garlic Oil (page 153)

1 pound flat iron steak

½ teaspoon sea salt

⅛ teaspoon freshly ground black pepper

1 teaspoon chili powder

6 scallions, green parts only, finely chopped

¼ cup freshly squeezed lime juice

8 corn tortillas

½ cup grated Cheddar cheese

SERVES 4 I love taco night at my house. I adore Mexican flavors, and the way they come together in these easy steak tacos is really fantastic. Use sirloin if you can't find flat iron steak. To make this dish IBS-C and GERD friendly, see the Tip.

1. In a large nonstick skillet over medium-high heat, heat the garlic oil until it shimmers.

2. Season the steak with the salt, pepper, and chili powder. Add it to the hot skillet and cook for about 5 minutes per side, or until your desired doneness. Transfer the steak to a cutting board and cut it against the grain into strips. Return the skillet to the heat.

3. Return the steak strips to the hot pan, and add the scallions and lime juice. Cook for 2 minutes.

4. Serve on the corn tortillas topped with the cheese.

COOKING TIP To cut steak against the grain, look at the meat and note the direction the long grains of the steak run. Cut perpendicular to this, which tenderizes the meat.

SUBSTITUTION TIP If you have IBS-C, omit the cheese. To make this GERD friendly, replace the garlic oil with 1 tablespoon olive oil and the chili powder with 1 teaspoon ground cumin. Omit the black pepper, lime juice, and scallions.

Per Serving (4 ounces meat, 2 tortillas, 2 tablespoons cheese) Calories: 460; Total Fat: 19g; Saturated Fat: 6; Carbohydrates: 24g; Fiber: 4g; Sodium: 408mg; Protein: 48g

Sirloin Chimichurri

5-INGREDIENT | 30-MINUTE | GLUTEN-FREE | LOW-CARB

SERVES 4 Chimichurri is not only delicious on chicken and beef. It's also wonderful combined with roasted root veggies. If you like, roast some red potatoes as a side dish and toss them with a few tablespoons of the chimichurri.

Prep: 5 minutes
Cook: 10 minutes

1 pound sirloin steak

½ teaspoon sea salt

⅛ teaspoon freshly ground black pepper

½ cup Chimichurri Sauce (page 158)

1. Preheat the broiler to high.

2. Season the sirloin with salt and pepper and place it on a broiling pan.

3. Broil the steak for about 4 minutes per side, or until your desired doneness.

4. Slice the steak into 1-inch-thick slices and serve topped with the chimichurri.

COOKING TIP Cut the steak against the grain to tenderize it.

Per Serving (4 ounces steak with 2 tablespoons chimichurri) Calories: 331; Total Fat: 19g; Saturated Fat: 4; Carbohydrates: 2g; Fiber: 4g; Sodium: 499mg; Protein: 35g

Flanken-Style Beef Ribs *with* Quick Slaw

5-INGREDIENT | 30-MINUTE | GLUTEN-FREE | LOW-CARB

Prep: 10 minutes
Cook: 8 minutes

1 pound flanken-style
beef ribs

½ teaspoon sea salt

⅛ teaspoon freshly ground
black pepper

2 tablespoons Garlic Oil
(page 153)

2 cups shredded cabbage

6 scallions, green parts only,
chopped

¼ cup Lemon-Dill Vinaigrette
(page 157)

SERVES 4 This is one of my go-to quick weeknight meals. I actually cook these ribs on my electric grill, which makes them cook even more quickly (in about 5 minutes), so, if you have one, feel free to use it in place of the skillet method recommended below. To make this GERD friendly, see the Tip.

1. Season the ribs with salt and pepper.

2. In a large nonstick skillet over medium-high heat, heat the garlic oil until it shimmers.

3. Add the ribs and cook for about 4 minutes per side, or until browned.

4. In a large bowl, combine the cabbage, scallions, and vinaigrette. Toss to combine.

INGREDIENT TIP Flanken-style beef ribs are long, thin-cut ribs that are crosscut through the bone. This cut is also commonly called Korean-style, and can be found at most Korean meat markets. If you don't see this cut on display at your local butcher, just ask them to prepare it for you.

SUBSTITUTION TIP To make this GERD friendly, omit the garlic oil and use 2 tablespoons olive oil instead. Omit the black pepper and the scallions, and use apple cider vinegar in the vinaigrette.

Per Serving (4 ounces ribs with ½ cup slaw) Calories: 357; Total Fat: 22g; Saturated Fat: 5; Carbohydrates: 4g; Fiber: 2g; Sodium: 319mg; Protein: 35g

Easy Shepherd's Pie

30-MINUTE | GLUTEN-FREE

SERVES 4 Instead of baking this shepherd's pie, you cook the filling and then quickly broil the potatoes to melt the cheese. With veggies, a starch, and a grain, this is an entire meal in one dish. To make this dish IBS-C and GERD friendly, see the Tip.

1. Heat the broiler to high.

2. In a large nonstick skillet over medium-high heat, heat the garlic oil until it shimmers.

3. Add the lamb and carrots. Cook for about 5 minutes, stirring, until the lamb is browned.

4. Stir in the broth, rosemary, salt, and pepper. Cook for 2 minutes more. Spoon the mixture into a 9-inch-square casserole.

5. Spread the mashed potatoes over the top and sprinkle with the cheese.

6. Broil the pie for about 3 minutes, watching closely, until the cheese melts.

SUBSTITUTION TIP If you have IBS-C, omit the cheese. To make this GERD friendly, omit the garlic oil (no need to replace it—it's just for flavor) and the black pepper and reduce the cheese to ¼ cup.

Per Serving (½ cup meat and veggies, ¼ cup potatoes) Calories: 577; Total Fat: 30g; Saturated Fat: 14; Carbohydrates: 38g; Fiber: 7g; Sodium: 490mg; Protein: 40g

Prep: 15 minutes
Cook: 10 minutes

2 tablespoons Garlic Oil (page 153)

1 pound ground lamb

2 carrots, chopped

¼ cup Low-FODMAP Poultry Broth (page 152)

1 tablespoon chopped fresh rosemary leaves

½ teaspoon sea salt

¼ teaspoon freshly ground black pepper

1 recipe Mashed Potatoes (page 54), hot

½ cup grated Cheddar cheese

Breaded Thin-Cut Pork Chops

5-INGREDIENT | 30-MINUTE | GLUTEN-FREE

Prep: 10 minutes
Cook: 20 minutes

2 cups gluten-free
bread crumbs

1 teaspoon dried thyme

1 teaspoon sea salt

¼ teaspoon freshly ground
black pepper

4 (4- to 6-ounce) thin-cut
pork chops

¼ cup Dijon mustard

SERVES 4 Thin-cut pork chops cook quickly in the oven, which makes them the perfect meal for when you're in a hurry. No need to get fancy with the sides here—a simple salad with your favorite low-FODMAP vinaigrette is satisfying but keeps carb counts low, if you're watching carbs. To make this GERD friendly, see the Tip.

1. Preheat the oven to 425°F.

2. In a small bowl, stir together the bread crumbs, thyme, salt, and pepper.

3. Spread the pork chops on both sides with mustard. Dip them into the seasoned bread crumbs to coat. Put the pork chops on a nonstick rimmed baking sheet.

4. Bake for about 20 minutes to an internal temperature of 165°F measured with a meat thermometer.

SUBSTITUTION TIP To make this GERD friendly, omit the black pepper and reduce the mustard to 2 tablespoons.

Per Serving (1 pork chop) Calories: 589; Total Fat: 32g; Saturated Fat: 11; Carbohydrates: 40g; Fiber: 3g; Sodium: 1,120mg; Protein: 33g

Pork Tenderloin Chops *with* Potatoes *and* Pan Sauce

5-INGREDIENT | GLUTEN-FREE | 30-MINUTE

SERVES 4 These simple pork tenderloin chops come together with a lovely pan sauce that coats the pork and potatoes, adding deep flavor. Serve with a side of steamed veggies, such as broccoli or broccolini for a full meal. To make this GERD friendly, see the Tip.

Prep: 10 minutes
Cook: 20 minutes

4 tablespoons garlic oil, divided

2 cups chopped Yukon Gold potatoes

1 teaspoon sea salt, divided

1 pound pork tenderloin, cut into 8 slices

½ teaspoon black pepper

1 cup low-FODMAP poultry broth (page 152)

3 tablespoons very cold butter, cut into pieces

¼ cup flat-leafed parsley leaves

1. In a large skillet, heat 2 tablespoons of the garlic oil on medium-high until they shimmer.

2. Add the potatoes and ½ teaspoon of the sea salt and cook, stirring occasionally, until they are soft and browned, about 10 minutes. Remove and set aside tented with foil to keep warm.

3. In the same pot, add the remaining 2 tablespoons of garlic oil. Season the pork tenderloin pieces with the remaining ½ teaspoon of sea salt and the pepper. Add to the hot oil and cook without moving until well browned on both sides, about 5 minutes per side.

4. Set aside tented with foil.

5. Add the poultry broth to the pan, using the side of the spoon to scrape any browned bits from the bottom of the pan. Reduce the heat to medium-low. Simmer until the liquid reduces by half.

6. Whisk in the butter one piece at a time until it is melted. Spoon the sauce over the potatoes and the meat. Garnish with the parsley leaves.

SUBSTITUTION TIP To make this GERD friendly, omit the black pepper, peppercorns, and the garlic oil. Use 4 tablespoons olive oil instead. For the broth, use 1 celery stalk instead of the leek.

Per Serving (4 ounces) Calories: 422; Total Fat: 27g; Saturated Fat: 9g; Carbohydrates: 12g; Fiber: 2g; Sodium: 791mg; Protein: 32g

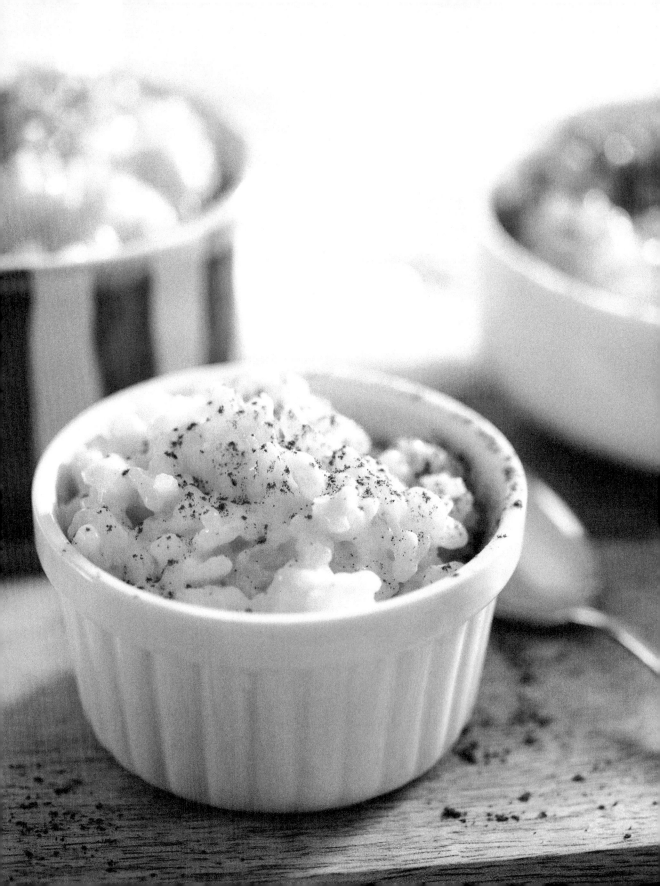

Snacks *and* Sweets

← *Coconut Pudding, page 144*

Prosciutto-Wrapped Cantaloupe

5-INGREDIENT | 30-MINUTE | GERD FRIENDLY | GLUTEN-FREE | LOW-CARB

Prep: 10 minutes
Cook: 0 minutes

8 (½- to 1-inch-thick)
cantaloupe wedges,
rind removed

8 thin prosciutto slices

SERVES 4 Prosciutto tastes delicious when paired with any type of melon. The result is a little salty, a little sweet, and a light, low-FODMAP snack. Substitute honeydew melon or casaba melon, which are both also low in FODMAPs, if you prefer. Avoid watermelon.

Wrap each melon wedge in a slice of prosciutto and secure it with a toothpick. Chill or serve immediately.

INGREDIENT TIP Look for prosciutto in the deli section of the grocery store. If you cannot find it, use thinly sliced Canadian bacon instead.

Per Serving (2 wedges) Calories: 73; Total Fat: 2g; Saturated Fat: <1g; Carbohydrates: 4g; Fiber: 0g; Sodium: 517mg; Protein: 9g

Cucumbers *with* Cottage Cheese Ranch Dip

30-MINUTE | GERD FRIENDLY | GLUTEN-FREE | VEGETARIAN

SERVES 4 This ranch dip is especially delicious with cucumber slices, as well as other low-FODMAP veggies, such as red bell peppers (my favorite) or sliced zucchini. Monash University notes that up to ¼ cup of cottage cheese won't raise your FODMAP load too high, so this is an easy and delicious snack you can enjoy any time. To make this IBS-C and Big 8 Allergen friendly, see the Tip.

In a medium bowl, stir together the cottage cheese, mayonnaise, scallions, dill, lemon zest, salt, and pepper until well mixed. Chill or serve immediately with the cucumber slices.

SUBSTITUTION TIP If you have IBS-C or are allergic or intolerant to dairy, replace the cottage cheese with ¼ cup nondairy plain yogurt, such as coconut yogurt.

Per Serving (½ cucumber with ¼ cup dip) Calories: 171; Total Fat: 11g; Saturated Fat: 2g; Carbohydrates: 15g; Fiber: 1g; Sodium: 565mg; Protein: 6g

Prep: 10 minutes
Cook: 0 minutes

½ cup cottage cheese

½ cup Low-FODMAP Mayonnaise (page 151)

6 scallions, green parts only, finely chopped

1 teaspoon chopped fresh dill

Zest of 1 lemon

½ teaspoon sea salt

¼ teaspoon freshly ground black pepper

2 cucumbers, sliced

Low-FODMAP Hummus

5-INGREDIENT | 30-MINUTE | GLUTEN-FREE | LOW-CARB | VEGAN

Prep: 10 minutes
Cook: 0 minutes

1 zucchini

2 tablespoons tahini

2 tablespoons Garlic Oil
(page 153)

Juice of 1 lemon

½ teaspoon sea salt

Assorted low-FODMAP
veggies, for dipping

SERVES 4 You'll need a blender or a food processor to make this hummus, which uses zucchini in place of the more traditional chickpeas. If you want that chickpea flavor, add up to ¼ cup chickpeas along with the zucchini, but proceed with caution, as chickpeas are a bit high in oligosaccharides. According to the Monash University Low-FODMAP Diet app, a ¼-cup serving per day may not cause issues. I actually prefer the dip made just with zucchini—it's one of my favorite snacks to serve with low-FODMAP veggies. To make this GERD friendly, see the Tip.

1. In a blender, combine the zucchini, tahini, garlic oil, lemon juice, and salt. Process until smooth.

2. Serve with the veggies for dipping.

SUBSTITUTION TIP To make this GERD friendly, omit the garlic oil and replace it with 2 tablespoons sesame oil. Omit the lemon juice and add ¼ cup water and the grated zest of 1 lemon along with ¼ cup chopped fresh parsley leaves.

Per Serving (about 2 tablespoons) Calories: 116; Total Fat: 11g; Saturated Fat: 2g; Carbohydrates: 4g; Fiber: 1g; Sodium: 251mg; Protein: 2g

Easy Trail Mix

5-INGREDIENT | 30-MINUTE | GERD FRIENDLY | GLUTEN-FREE | LOW-CARB | VEGAN

SERVES 4 This recipe contains small amounts of certain foods (like dried cranberries) that won't overload you with FODMAPs provided you exercise portion control. So, for dried cranberries, you can safely have 1 tablespoon; for dried bananas, you can have about 20 chips (about ½ cup); for almonds, you can have about 10 nuts (2 tablespoons); and for peanuts, you can have about ¼ cup. To make this Big 8 Allergen friendly, see the Tip.

In a small bowl, mix all the ingredients. Store in a resealable bag at room temperature for up to 1 month.

SUBSTITUTION TIP If you are allergic to peanuts and tree nuts, replace them with ½ cup pumpkin seeds and ¼ cup sunflower seeds.

Per Serving (about ¼ cup) Calories: 158; Total Fat: 11g; Saturated Fat: 1g; Carbohydrates: 13g; Fiber: 4g; Sodium: 2mg; Protein: 5g

Prep: 10 minutes
Cook: 0 minutes

1 cup dried bananas

½ cup raw unsalted almonds

¼ cup raw unsalted peanuts

¼ cup dried cranberries

Deviled Eggs

5-INGREDIENT | 30-MINUTE | GLUTEN-FREE | LOW-CARB | VEGETARIAN

Prep: 10 minutes
Cook: 0 minutes

6 hardboiled eggs, peeled and halved lengthwise

½ cup Low-FODMAP Mayonnaise (page 151)

2 tablespoons Dijon mustard

3 scallions, green parts only, minced

½ teaspoon sea salt

½ teaspoon ground paprika

⅛ teaspoon freshly ground black pepper

SERVES 6 Buying peeled hardboiled eggs from the deli or egg section makes this recipe a snap. You can make these ahead and take them for snacks on the go. If you prefer to boil your own eggs, see the Tip for instructions, as well as for a GERD friendly variation.

1. Into a small bowl, scoop the egg yolks from the whites. Set the whites aside.

2. Add the mayonnaise, mustard, scallions, salt, paprika, and pepper to the yolks and mash them with a fork.

3. Spoon the mixture back into the egg whites.

COOKING TIP To hardboil eggs, place the eggs in a single layer in a large saucepan. Add enough water to cover the eggs by 1 inch. Put the pan over medium-high heat and bring to a boil. Boil for 1 minute. Turn off the heat, cover the pan, and let the eggs sit for 14 minutes. Run the eggs under cold water to stop the cooking.

SUBSTITUTION TIP To make this GERD friendly, omit the paprika, black pepper, and scallions and add 1 tablespoon chopped fresh dill.

Per Serving (2 halves) Calories: 240; Total Fat: 18g; Saturated Fat: 4g; Carbohydrates: 11g; Fiber: 1g; Sodium: 537mg; Protein: 10g

Parmesan Potato Wedges

5-INGREDIENT | GLUTEN-FREE | VEGETARIAN

SERVES 4 If you like French fries, you'll enjoy these flavorful, aromatic baked potato wedges. These make a tasty snack or a delicious side dish with a fish, chicken, or beef main course. For the best results, serve immediately and do not reheat. To make this IBS-C and GERD friendly, see the Tip.

1. Preheat the oven to 425°F.

2. In a small bowl, combine the potatoes, garlic oil, Parmesan cheese, salt, and pepper and toss to coat the potatoes with the cheese and oil. Spread the potatoes in a single layer on a rimmed baking sheet.

3. Bake for about 25 minutes, or until the potatoes are tender.

Prep: 10 minutes
Cook: 25 minutes

4 red potatoes,
cut into wedges

2 tablespoons Garlic Oil
(page 153)

¼ cup grated Parmesan
cheese

½ teaspoon sea salt

¼ teaspoon freshly ground
black pepper

SUBSTITUTION TIP If you have IBS-C, omit the cheese. To make this GERD friendly, replace the garlic oil with 1 tablespoon olive oil. Omit the black pepper, and reduce the cheese to 2 tablespoons.

Per Serving (1 potato) Calories: 232; Total Fat: 9g; Saturated Fat: 2g; Carbohydrates: 34g; Fiber: 4g; Sodium: 313mg; Protein: 6g

Peanut Butter Cookies

5-INGREDIENT | 30-MINUTE | GERD FRIENDLY | GLUTEN-FREE | LOW-CARB | VEGETARIAN

Prep: 15 minutes
Cook: 10 minutes

1 cup sugar-free natural peanut butter

½ cup packed brown sugar

1 egg, beaten

1 teaspoon baking soda

½ teaspoon vanilla extract

Pinch sea salt

MAKES 24 These peanut butter cookies are easy and delicious. Because they call for only a few ingredients, prep takes no time at all and you can have warm, smile-inducing treats in about 30 minutes. The recipe is deliberately flourless. For a little variety, add ¼ cup dark chocolate chips. If you have GERD, skip the chocolate. To make these cookies Big 8 Allergen friendly, see the Tip.

1. Preheat the oven to 350°F.
2. Line a baking sheet with parchment paper and set it aside.
3. In a medium bowl, mix the peanut butter and brown sugar.
4. Stir in the egg, baking soda, vanilla, and salt until well combined. Roll the dough into 24 teaspoon-size balls and place them on the prepared sheet. Flatten slightly with a fork in a crosshatch pattern.
5. Bake for about 10 minutes, or until the cookies puff and turn golden brown.

SUBSTITUTION TIP If you are allergic to peanuts, replace the peanut butter with 1 cup almond butter.

Per Serving (1 cookie) Calories: 78; Total Fat: 6g; Saturated Fat: 1g; Carbohydrates: 5g; Fiber: <1g; Sodium: 113mg; Protein: 3g

No-Bake Chocolate Cookies

5-INGREDIENT | 30-MINUTE | GLUTEN-FREE | VEGETARIAN

MAKES 15 These were one of my favorite cookies to make when I was a child. I love the combination of the almond butter, chocolate, and oatmeal, and they cool quickly (meaning you can eat them very quickly!), especially if you put them in the refrigerator or freezer. To make these cookies Big 8 Allergen friendly, see the Tip.

Prep: 10 minutes
Cook: 5 minutes
Cooling: 10 to 20 minutes

1 cup sugar

½ cup unsweetened almond milk

2 tablespoons unsweetened cocoa powder

1½ cups quick-cooking oatmeal

¾ cup almond butter

1 teaspoon vanilla extract

Pinch sea salt

1. Line a baking sheet with parchment paper and set it aside.

2. In a large saucepan over high heat, stir together the sugar, almond milk, and cocoa powder. Bring the mixture to a boil and boil for 1 minute, stirring constantly.

3. Remove the pan from the heat and immediately stir in the oatmeal, almond butter, vanilla, and salt. Spoon 1-tablespoon portions onto the prepared sheet.

4. Refrigerate for 20 minutes or freeze for 10 minutes to cool.

SUBSTITUTION TIP If you are allergic to tree nuts, replace the almond butter with ½ cup sugar-free natural peanut butter.

Per Serving (2 cookies) Calories: 107; Total Fat: 3g; Saturated Fat: 2g; Carbohydrates: 20g; Fiber: 1g; Sodium: 14mg; Protein: 2g

Chocolate-Peanut Butter Balls

5-INGREDIENT | 30-MINUTE | GLUTEN-FREE | VEGETARIAN

Prep: 10 minutes
Cook: 5 minutes

½ cup sugar-free natural peanut butter

¼ cup unsalted butter, at room temperature

1 cup confectioners' sugar

1 cup semi-sweet chocolate chips

2 tablespoons coconut oil

MAKES 16 This is another of my favorite childhood recipes. It's also something I make for my family every Christmas, and always have. After dipping the balls in chocolate, chill them in the freezer for about 10 minutes so the chocolate shell hardens. These freeze well, too. To make these treats Big 8 Allergen friendly, see the Tip.

1. Line a baking sheet with parchment paper and set it aside.

2. In a large bowl, stir together the peanut butter, butter, and confectioners' sugar until well mixed. Form the mixture into about 16 tablespoon-size balls.

3. In a medium saucepan over low heat, melt the chocolate chips and coconut oil for about 5 minutes, stirring constantly until melted and smooth.

4. Dip the balls in the chocolate mixture and place on the prepared sheet. Freeze for 10 minutes to set the chocolate coating.

SUBSTITUTION TIP If you are allergic to peanuts, substitute ½ cup almond butter for the peanut butter.

Per Serving (2 balls) Calories: 165; Total Fat: 11g; Saturated Fat: 5g; Carbohydrates: 15g; Fiber: <1g; Sodium: 92mg; Protein: 2g

Chocolate-Chia Pudding

5-INGREDIENT | GLUTEN-FREE | VEGAN

SERVES 6 Chia seeds plump and turn into gel-like globes (similar to tapioca) when added to liquid so they make a great pudding thickener. They are also an excellent source of omega-3 fatty acids. To make this GERD friendly, see the Tip.

Prep: 10 minutes
Cook: 5 minutes
Chilling: Overnight

2 cups unsweetened almond milk

½ cup pure maple syrup

3 tablespoons unsweetened cocoa powder

½ teaspoon vanilla extract

½ cup chia seeds

1. In a medium saucepan over medium heat, combine the almond milk, maple syrup, cocoa powder, and vanilla. Cook just until the cocoa powder dissolves, whisking constantly.

2. Remove the pan from heat and let cool slightly. Stir in the chia seeds.

3. Refrigerate overnight.

SUBSTITUTION TIP To make this GERD friendly, turn it into a maple-chia pudding—omit the cocoa powder.

Per Serving (about ½ cup) Calories: 273; Total Fat: 20g; Saturated Fat: 17g; Carbohydrates: 24g; Fiber: 4g; Sodium: 15mg; Protein: 3g

Coconut Pudding

5-INGREDIENT | GLUTEN-FREE | LOW-CARB | VEGAN

Prep: 10 minutes
Cook: 5 minutes
Chilling: 2 hours or overnight

2 cups coconut milk

4 packets stevia

3 tablespoons water

3 tablespoons cornstarch

⅛ teaspoon sea salt

¼ cup unsweetened toasted coconut

SERVES 4 While this pudding cooks quickly, you'll need to chill it for a few hours unless you enjoy your pudding warm. It's a delicious dessert to prepare in the morning and refrigerate through the day so you can come home to a tasty sweet treat to enjoy after dinner. To make this GERD friendly, see the Tip.

1. In a medium saucepan over medium-high heat, combine the coconut milk and stevia. Bring to a boil, stirring constantly.

2. In a small bowl, whisk the water and cornstarch. In a thin stream, pour this slurry into the boiling coconut milk, whisking constantly. Continue to cook the pudding for about 3 minutes more, until it starts to thicken.

3. Whisk in the salt.

4. Divide the pudding among four dessert dishes. Top with the coconut. Chill for at least 2 hours.

SUBSTITUTION TIP To make this GERD friendly, replace the coconut milk with 2 cups light coconut milk and omit the toasted coconut.

Per Serving (½ cup) Calories: 317; Total Fat: 30g; Saturated Fat: 27g; Carbohydrates: 13g; Fiber: 3g; Sodium: 78mg; Protein: 3g

Rice Pudding

5-INGREDIENT | 30-MINUTE | GERD FRIENDLY | GLUTEN-FREE | LOW-CARB | VEGETARIAN

SERVES 4 Serve this pudding by itself or topped with Raspberry Sauce (page 165). I adore pudding, and I have since I was a child. It's easy to adapt the recipe to the flavors you like, as well as to numerous diets like a low-carb diet or a low-FODMAP diet. To make this Big 8 Allergen friendly, see the Tip.

Prep: 10 minutes
Cook: 17 minutes

2 cups unsweetened almond milk, divided

1½ cups cooked white rice

⅓ cup sugar

Pinch sea salt

1 egg, beaten

½ teaspoon vanilla extract

Freshly grated nutmeg, for garnishing (optional)

1. In a medium saucepan over medium heat, stir together 1½ cups almond milk, the rice, sugar, and salt. Cover and cook for about 15 minutes, or until thick.

2. Add the remaining ½ cup almond milk and the egg. Cook for 2 minutes, stirring constantly.

3. Remove the pan from the heat and stir in the vanilla.

4. Serve warm garnished with freshly grated nutmeg (if using).

SUBSTITUTION TIP If you're allergic to tree nuts, replace the almond milk with 2 cups lactose-free milk.

Per Serving (about ½ cup) Calories: 49; Total Fat: 2g; Saturated Fat: 0g; Carbohydrates: 7g; Fiber: <1g; Sodium: 91mg; Protein: <1g

Kiwi Yogurt Freezer Bars

5-INGREDIENT | GERD FRIENDLY | GLUTEN-FREE | LOW-CARB | VEGETARIAN

Prep: 10 minutes
Cook: 0 minutes
Freezing: Overnight

2 cups unsweetened
almond milk

4 kiwis, peeled and chopped

½ cup lactose-free
plain yogurt

4 packets stevia

SERVES 6 While I've chosen kiwi here as the primary fruit, you can use any low-FODMAP fruit you prefer, such as melons or strawberries, to make these delicious, creamy freezer treats. These need to freeze overnight, so plan to make them a day ahead.

1. In a blender, combine the almond milk, kiwis, yogurt, and stevia. Process until smooth.

2. Pour the mixture into 6 ice pop molds.

3. Refrigerate overnight.

INGREDIENT TIP If you don't have ice pop molds, use small (4-ounce) paper cups instead. Pour the mixture into the paper cups and cover them with aluminum foil. Insert ice pop sticks through the foil and freeze as directed.

Per Serving (1 bar) Calories: 59; Total Fat: 2g; Saturated Fat: 0g; Carbohydrates: 10g; Fiber: 2g; Sodium: 76mg; Protein: 2g

Banana Ice Cream

5-INGREDIENT | 30-MINUTE | GERD FRIENDLY | GLUTEN-FREE | VEGAN

PSERVES 2 This is the easiest ice cream ever—and it's pretty tasty to boot. It turns out frozen bananas are super creamy when you mash them in a blender with a little sweetener. I like to add a bit of cinnamon or nutmeg for extra flavor, but you can also add ginger, allspice, or any other spice.

Prep: 10 minutes
Cook: 0 minutes

3 bananas, peeled and frozen

3 packets stevia

¼ teaspoon ground nutmeg

In a blender or food processor, combine the bananas, stevia, and nutmeg. Blend until smooth.

INGREDIENT TIP This is a good use for very ripe bananas, so, if you have some, peel them and freeze for a quick dessert.

Per Serving (about ½ cup) Calories: 106; Total Fat: <1g; Saturated Fat: 0g; Carbohydrates: 27g; Fiber: 3g; Sodium: 1mg; Protein: 1g

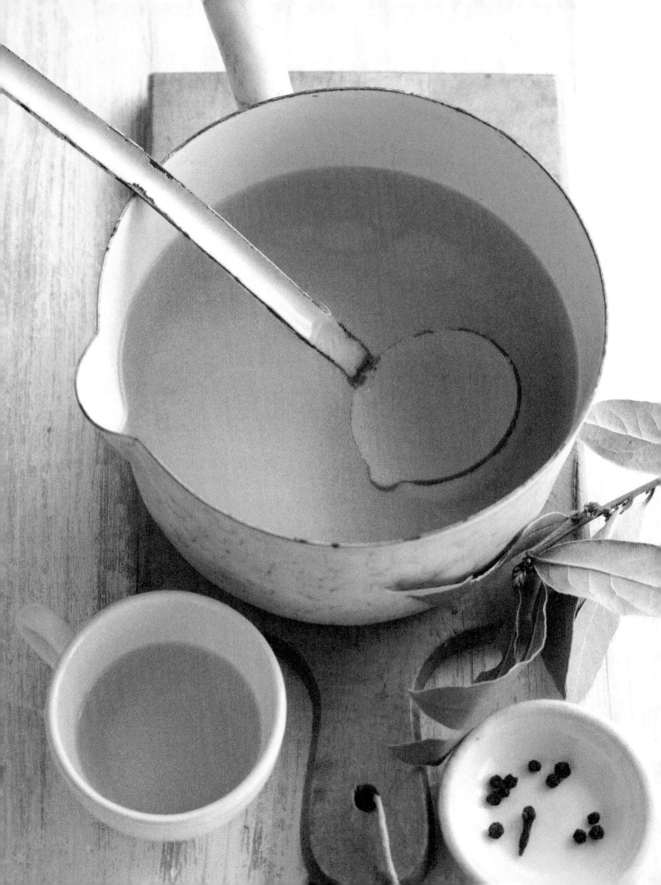

Broths, Sauces, *and* Condiments

← *Low-FODMAP Poultry Broth, page 152*

Low-FODMAP Vegetable Broth

5-INGREDIENT | GLUTEN-FREE | LOW-CARB | VEGAN

Prep: 10 minutes
Cook: 3 to 8 hours

3 carrots, roughly chopped

2 leeks, green parts only, roughly chopped

1 fennel bulb, roughly chopped

8 peppercorns

1 fresh rosemary sprig

MAKES 8 TO 10 CUPS If you have a large (8-quart) slow cooker, I recommend using it because it is the most hands-off way to make this nourishing, flavorful broth. You can also make this in a large stockpot on your stove top. The slow cooker will have less evaporation than the stove top method. This broth is made without salt so you can add seasonings to taste in your finished soups, stews, and other recipes. To make this GERD friendly, see the Tip.

1. In a large stockpot or slow cooker, combine the carrots, leeks, fennel, peppercorns, and rosemary.

2. Fill the pot about ¾ full, with enough water to cover the ingredients.

If using a stockpot: Place the pot over medium-low heat and bring the liquid to a simmer. Simmer for 3 hours.

If using a slow cooker: Cover the cooker, set the temperature to low, and cook for 8 hours.

3. Strain and discard the solids. Refrigerate or freeze the stock in 1-cup servings. The broth will keep in the refrigerator for about 5 days or in the freezer for up to 12 months.

SUBSTITUTION TIP To make this GERD friendly, omit the peppercorns and leeks. Add 1 celery stalk, roughly chopped.

Per Serving (1 cup) Calories: 15; Total Fat: 0g; Saturated Fat: 0g; Carbohydrates: 5g; Fiber: 0g; Sodium: 30mg; Protein: <1g

Low-FODMAP Mayonnaise

5-INGREDIENT | 30-MINUTE | GLUTEN-FREE | LOW-CARB | VEGETARIAN

MAKES ABOUT 1 CUP Commercial mayonnaise often contains high fructose corn syrup, which is most definitely not FODMAP friendly. Making your own mayonnaise doesn't take long, and it's a breeze if you use a food processor, blender, or immersion blender to make it. *If you are concerned about pathogens in raw egg yolks, use pasteurized eggs.* To make this GERD friendly, see the Tip.

Prep: 5 minutes
Cook: 0 minutes

1 egg yolk

1 tablespoon red wine vinegar

½ teaspoon Dijon mustard

¼ teaspoon sea salt

¾ cup extra-virgin olive oil

1. In a blender or food processor, combine the egg yolk, vinegar, mustard, and salt. Process for about 30 seconds until well combined. With a rubber spatula, scrape down the sides of the blender jar or food processor bowl.

2. Turn the blender or processor to medium speed. Very slowly, drip in the olive oil, 1 drop at a time as the processor or blender runs. After about 10 drops, leave the blender or processor running, then add the rest of the olive oil in a thin stream until it is incorporated and emulsified.

3. The mayo will keep refrigerated for up to 5 days.

SUBSTITUTION TIP If you have GERD, make this mayonnaise recipe variation, which doesn't contain vinegar. In a small bowl, whisk 1 egg yolk and 1 teaspoon Dijon mustard. Slowly, in a very thin stream, add 1 cup of olive oil, whisking the entire time. Whisk in 1 cup plain nonfat yogurt and season with ½ teaspoon salt.

Per Serving (2 tablespoons) Calories: 169; Total Fat: 20g; Saturated Fat: 3g; Carbohydrates: <1g; Fiber: 0g; Sodium: 63mg; Protein: <1g

Low-FODMAP Poultry Broth
or Meat Broth

5-INGREDIENT | GLUTEN-FREE | LOW-CARB

Prep: 10 minutes
Cook: 3 to 8 hours

3 pounds meaty bones

3 carrots, roughly chopped

2 leeks, green parts only, roughly chopped

8 peppercorns

1 fresh thyme sprig

MAKES 8 TO 10 CUPS This is a generic recipe you can use for any type of poultry or meat broth. The slow cooker method is the most hands off; if you don't have an 8-quart slow cooker, use a large stockpot on your stove top. Choose meaty bones, such as oxtails, turkey or chicken necks, backs, and wings, etc. To make this GERD friendly, see the Tip.

1. In a large stockpot or slow cooker, combine the bones, carrots, leeks, peppercorns, and thyme.

2. Fill the pot about ¾ full, with enough water to cover the ingredients.

If using a stockpot: Place the pot over medium-low heat and bring the liquid to a simmer. Simmer for 3 hours.

If using a slow cooker: Cover the cooker, set the temperature to low, and cook for 8 hours.

3. Strain and discard the solids.

4. Refrigerate the broth overnight. Skim the fat from the surface and discard.

5. Refrigerate or freeze the stock in 1-cup servings. The broth will keep in the refrigerator for about 5 days or in the freezer for up to 12 months.

SUBSTITUTION TIP To make this GERD friendly, omit the peppercorns and leeks. Add 1 celery stalk, roughly chopped.

Per Serving (1 cup): Calories: 15; Total Fat: 0g; Saturated Fat: 0g; Carbohydrates: 1.5g; Fiber: 0g; Sodium: 60mg; Protein: 1.5g

Garlic Oil

5-INGREDIENT | 30-MINUTE | GLUTEN-FREE | LOW-CARB | VEGAN

MAKES ⅓ CUP Making garlic-infused oil allows you to add the flavor of garlic to your foods without the FODMAPs that come from eating garlic. You can also make this oil with onions. It's important to strain out the garlic or onions before adding the oil to your foods. It will keep for about 5 days, so making small batches as you need them is best.

Prep: 5 minutes
Cook: 10 minutes

½ cup extra-virgin olive oil

5 garlic cloves, smashed

1. In a small saucepan over medium-low heat, combine the olive oil and garlic. Heat for 10 minutes, just barely simmering.

2. Strain and discard the garlic.

3. Store the oil in an airtight container in a dark cupboard.

COOKING TIP To make onion oil, substitute ½ onion, chopped, for the garlic. You can also make garlic and onion oil with ½ onion, 5 garlic cloves, smashed, and ½ cup extra-virgin olive oil.

Per Serving (1 tablespoon) Calories: 120; Total Fat: 14g; Saturated Fat: 2g; Carbohydrates: 0g; Fiber: 0g; Sodium: 0mg; Protein: 0g

Cilantro-Lime Vinaigrette

5-INGREDIENT | 30-MINUTE | GLUTEN-FREE | LOW-CARB | VEGAN

Prep: 10 minutes
Cook: 0 minutes

2 tablespoons freshly
squeezed lime juice

2 tablespoons Garlic Oil
(page 153)

¼ cup extra-virgin olive oil

¼ teaspoon sea salt

2 tablespoons chopped
fresh cilantro leaves

MAKES ½ CUP This is a refreshing, tangy vinaigrette that is delicious on salads, and equally tasty on chicken or fish. People with GERD can typically have about 1 tablespoon of vinaigrette safely. This will keep, refrigerated, for up to 5 days. To make this GERD friendly, see the Tip.

In a small bowl, whisk together the lime juice, garlic oil, olive oil, salt, and cilantro. Whisk again just before serving.

SUBSTITUTION TIP To make this GERD friendly, omit the garlic oil and reduce the serving size to 1 tablespoon.

Per Serving (2 tablespoons) Calories: 170; Total Fat: 20g; Saturated Fat: 3g; Carbohydrates: <1g; Fiber: 0g; Sodium: 119mg; Protein: <1g

Italian Basil Vinaigrette

5-INGREDIENT | 30-MINUTE | GLUTEN-FREE | LOW-CARB | VEGAN

MAKES ABOUT ½ CUP I love fresh basil. I adore the way it tastes and its aroma. It's delicious added to a salad or a gluten-free pasta salad, and its brightness immediately perks up even the most mundane foods. This basil vinaigrette will keep refrigerated for up to 5 days, so make it in small batches. To make this GERD friendly, see the Tip.

In a small bowl, whisk together all the ingredients. Whisk again just before serving.

SUBSTITUTION TIP To make this GERD friendly, replace the garlic oil with an equal amount of extra-virgin olive oil. Omit the black pepper and reduce the serving size to 1 tablespoon.

Per Serving (2 tablespoons) Calories: 124; Total Fat: 14g; Saturated Fat: 2g; Carbohydrates: <1g; Fiber: 0g; Sodium: 118mg; Protein: <1g

Prep: 10 minutes
Cook: 0 minutes

2 tablespoons apple cider vinegar

2 tablespoons extra-virgin olive oil

2 tablespoons Garlic Oil (page 153)

2 tablespoons chopped fresh basil leaves

½ teaspoon Dijon mustard

¼ teaspoon sea salt

⅛ teaspoon freshly ground black pepper

Balsamic Vinaigrette

5-INGREDIENT | 30-MINUTE | GLUTEN-FREE | LOW-CARB | VEGAN

Prep: 10 minutes
Cook: 0 minutes

2 tablespoons balsamic vinegar

1 tablespoon freshly squeezed orange juice

½ teaspoon grated orange zest

½ teaspoon Dijon mustard

⅓ cup extra-virgin olive oil

¼ teaspoon sea salt

⅛ teaspoon freshly ground black pepper

MAKES ABOUT ½ CUP Balsamic vinegar has a lovely sweetness to it as well as a heady aroma. I like it plain, just drizzled on foods, but it's really good in this vinaigrette, too. It will keep refrigerated for up to 5 days, so make it fresh as you need it. To make this GERD friendly, see the Tip.

In a small bowl, whisk together all the ingredients. Whisk again just before serving.

SUBSTITUTION TIP To make this GERD friendly, replace the orange juice with 1 additional tablespoon balsamic vinegar. Omit the black pepper and reduce the serving size to 1 tablespoon.

Per Serving (2 tablespoons) Calories: 146; Total Fat: 17g; Saturated Fat: 2g; Carbohydrates: <1g; Fiber: 0g; Sodium: 117mg; Protein: <1g

Lemon-Dill Vinaigrette

5-INGREDIENT | 30-MINUTE | GLUTEN-FREE | LOW-CARB | VEGAN

MAKES ABOUT ½ CUP The combination of lemon and dill is especially nice with fish and shellfish, so this makes a delicious vinaigrette for a salad to accompany a seafood main course. It's also a delicious topping for fish or tossed with steamed vegetables. It will keep refrigerated for up to 5 days. To make this GERD friendly, see the Tip.

In a small bowl, whisk together all the ingredients. Whisk again just before serving.

SUBSTITUTION TIP To make this GERD friendly, replace the lemon juice with 3 tablespoons apple cider vinegar. Replace the garlic oil with ¼ cup extra-virgin olive oil. Omit the black pepper and reduce the serving size to 1 tablespoon.

Per Serving (2 tablespoons) Calories: 128; Total Fat: 14g; Saturated Fat: 2g; Carbohydrates: 1g; Fiber: 0g; Sodium: 130mg; Protein: <1g

Prep: 10 minutes
Cook: 0 minutes

¼ cup Garlic Oil (page 153)

3 tablespoons freshly squeezed lemon juice

½ teaspoon grated lemon zest

2 tablespoons chopped fresh dill

½ teaspoon Dijon mustard

¼ teaspoon sea salt

⅛ teaspoon freshly ground black pepper

Chimichurri Sauce

30-MINUTE | GLUTEN-FREE | LOW-CARB | VEGAN

Prep: 10 minutes
Cook: 0 minutes

½ cup red wine vinegar

¼ cup extra-virgin olive oil

2 tablespoons Garlic Oil
(page 153)

¼ cup parsley leaves,
finely chopped

Zest of 1 lemon

Juice of 1 lemon

½ teaspoon sea salt

⅛ teaspoon red pepper flakes

⅛ teaspoon freshly ground
black pepper

MAKES 1 CUP Chimichurri sauce has its roots in South America, and is a staple of Argentinean cuisine. This unique and fresh-tasting sauce, which requires no cooking, is especially delicious on steak and other red meats—try it on a hamburger, for instance. Refrigerate it for up to 5 days, or freeze it in ¼-cup amounts tightly sealed for up to 6 months.

In a small bowl, whisk together all the ingredients. Whisk again just before serving.

COOKING TIP The best tool for zesting a lemon is a rasp-style grater. As you zest the lemon, avoid the white part underneath the peel (the pith) because it is bitter.

Per Serving (2 tablespoons) Calories: 90; Total Fat: 10g; Saturated Fat: 1g; Carbohydrates: <1g; Fiber: 0g; Sodium: 120mg; Protein: <1g

Macadamia Spinach Pesto

30-MINUTE | GLUTEN-FREE | LOW-CARB | VEGETARIAN

MAKES ABOUT 1 CUP I love this tangy twist on pesto. It's fantastic on gluten-free pasta, or on hot zucchini noodles. It is also delicious with eggs or spooned as a sauce over a protein. Freeze leftovers in ¼-cup portions for later use. To make this IBS-C and GERD friendly, see the Tip.

In a blender or food processor, combine all the ingredients. Process until everything is well chopped and combined.

SUBSTITUTION TIP If you have IBS-C, make the pesto without the cheese or avoid using this recipe. To make this GERD friendly, replace the garlic oil with an equal amount of olive oil. Reduce the serving size to 1 tablespoon.

Per Serving (2 tablespoons) Calories: 115; Total Fat: 12g; Saturated Fat: 2g; Carbohydrates: 1g; Fiber: <1g; Sodium: 189mg; Protein: 3g

Prep: 10 minutes
Cook: 0 minutes

2 cups fresh baby spinach

½ cup fresh basil leaves

½ cup grated Parmesan cheese

¼ cup Garlic Oil (page 153)

¼ cup macadamia nuts

Zest of 1 lemon

½ teaspoon sea salt

Homemade Barbecue Sauce

30-MINUTE | GLUTEN-FREE | LOW-CARB | VEGAN

Prep: 10 minutes
Cook: 10 minutes

6 scallions, green parts only, minced

½ cup apple cider vinegar

2 tablespoons Garlic Oil (page 153)

2 tablespoons tomato paste

1 teaspoon liquid smoke

1 packet stevia

1 teaspoon chili powder

½ teaspoon sea salt

⅛ teaspoon freshly ground black pepper

MAKES ABOUT 1 CUP This smoky barbecue sauce is delicious on grilled meats or as a tasty dip for veggies or fries. Try combining it with a few tablespoons of Low-FODMAP Mayonnaise (page 151) for a creamy, smoky dip.

1. In a small saucepan over medium heat, combine all the ingredients.

2. Simmer for 5 minutes, stirring. Refrigerate any leftovers for up to 5 days.

INGREDIENT TIP You can find liquid smoke with the sauces and condiments in the grocery store. A little goes a long way, so start with a small amount and taste and adjust as you work to determine your preferred level of smokiness.

Per Serving (2 tablespoons) Calories: 41; Total Fat: 4g; Saturated Fat: 0g; Carbohydrates: 2g; Fiber: <1g; Sodium: 127mg; Protein: <1g

Stir-Fry Sauce

5-INGREDIENT | 30-MINUTE | GLUTEN-FREE | LOW-CARB | VEGAN

MAKES ABOUT ½ CUP Use this Asian-inspired stir-fry sauce with meat or veggie recipes such as Vegetable Stir-Fry (page 78). This will keep refrigerated for up to 5 days. To make this GERD friendly, see the Tip.

In a small bowl, whisk together the orange juice, soy sauce, cornstarch, ginger, and red pepper flakes.

COOKING TIP Whisk this again just before adding it to your stir-fry to incorporate any cornstarch that settled to the bottom, to prevent it from getting grainy or lumpy.

SUBSTITUTION TIP To make this GERD friendly, omit the orange juice and replace it with ¼ cup water and the grated zest of 1 orange.

Prep: 5 minutes
Cook: 0 minutes

¼ cup freshly squeezed orange juice

3 tablespoons gluten-free soy sauce

2 tablespoons cornstarch

1 tablespoon peeled and grated fresh ginger

Pinch red pepper flakes

Per Serving (2 tablespoons) Calories: 33; Total Fat: <1g; Saturated Fat: 0g; Carbohydrates: 7g; Fiber: 0g; Sodium: 677mg; Protein: 1g

Sweet-and-Sour Sauce

30-MINUTE | GLUTEN-FREE | LOW-CARB | VEGAN

Prep: 5 minutes
Cook: 5 minutes

½ cup pineapple juice

⅓ cup rice vinegar

¼ cup packed brown sugar

¼ cup tomato sauce

1 tablespoon gluten-free soy sauce

1 tablespoon cornstarch

MAKES ABOUT 1 CUP If you enjoy Chinese takeout, you'll love this sauce. It's especially good on chicken or shrimp. You can make it ahead of time if you wish—it will keep refrigerated for up to 5 days.

1. In a small saucepan over medium-high heat, whisk together all the ingredients.

2. Simmer for about 5 minutes, whisking, until the sauce thickens.

INGREDIENT TIP If you can't find rice vinegar, use an equal amount of white vinegar instead.

Per Serving (2 tablespoons) Calories: 39; Total Fat: 0g; Saturated Fat: 0g; Carbohydrates: 8g; Fiber: 0g; Sodium: 155mg; Protein: <1g

Teriyaki Sauce

5-INGREDIENT | 30-MINUTE | GLUTEN-FREE | LOW-CARB | VEGAN

MAKES ABOUT 1 CUP Teriyaki sauce is sweet, salty, and a little sticky—and it's fantastic on chicken, fish, turkey, or beef. I enjoy teriyaki sauce on rice and steamed veggies as well. This will keep refrigerated for up to 5 days. To make this GERD friendly, see the Tip.

Prep: 5 minutes
Cook: 5 minutes

½ cup water

½ cup gluten-free soy sauce

¼ cup packed brown sugar

2 tablespoons mirin

1 tablespoon Garlic Oil (page 153)

1 tablespoon peeled and grated fresh ginger

1. In a small saucepan over medium-high heat, whisk together all the ingredients.

2. Simmer for about 5 minutes, whisking, until the sauce thickens.

SUBSTITUTION TIP To make this GERD friendly, omit the garlic oil.

INGREDIENT TIP If you can't find mirin, replace it with an equal amount of rice vinegar or white vinegar.

Per Serving (2 tablespoons) Calories: 52; Total Fat: 2g; Saturated Fat: 0g; Carbohydrates: 8g; Fiber: 0g; Sodium: 1,040mg; Protein: 2g

Olive Tapenade

30-MINUTE | GLUTEN-FREE | LOW-CARB

Prep: 5 minutes
Cook: 0 minutes

1 cup chopped black olives

2 tablespoons Garlic Oil
(page 153)

2 tablespoons chopped
fresh basil leaves

1 anchovy fillet, minced

1 tablespoon capers, chopped

Juice of ½ lemon

½ teaspoon sea salt

⅛ teaspoon freshly ground
black pepper

MAKES ABOUT 1 CUP This versatile olive tapenade is a tasty sandwich spread, a delicious topper for fish, beef, or chicken, or a lovely dip for veggies. For the best flavor, use the best black olives you can afford. To make this GERD friendly, see the Tip.

In a small bowl, stir together all the ingredients until well mixed.

SUBSTITUTION TIP To make this GERD friendly, replace the garlic oil with 2 tablespoons olive oil. Omit the lemon juice and black pepper and add the grated zest of ½ lemon.

Per Serving (2 tablespoons) Calories: 61; Total Fat: 6g; Saturated Fat: <1g; Carbohydrates: 2g; Fiber: <1g; Sodium: 388mg; Protein: <1g

Raspberry Sauce

5-INGREDIENT | 30-MINUTE | GLUTEN-FREE | VEGAN

SERVES 4 Serve this fresh and fruity sauce over Coconut Pudding (page 144), Rice Pudding (page 145), Chocolate-Chia Pudding (page 143), or a scoop of lactose-free ice cream. It's even delicious added to a smoothie. To make this GERD friendly, see the Tip.

Prep: 5 minutes
Cook: 10 minutes

1 cup fresh raspberries

¼ cup sugar

2 tablespoons water

1. In a large saucepan over medium-high heat, cook the raspberries, sugar, and water, stirring frequently and mashing the raspberries with a spoon. Bring to a boil. Reduce the heat to low and simmer for 5 minutes.

2. Strain the sauce through a fine-mesh sieve to remove the seeds. Chill before serving.

SUBSTITUTION TIP Raspberries tend to be a little acidic, so they might irritate GERD. If this is a problem for you, use fresh strawberries, which are less acidic, in place of the raspberries.

Per Serving (about 2 tablespoons) Calories: 63; Total Fat: 0g; Saturated Fat: 0g; Carbohydrates: 16g; Fiber: 2g; Sodium: 1mg; Protein: <1g

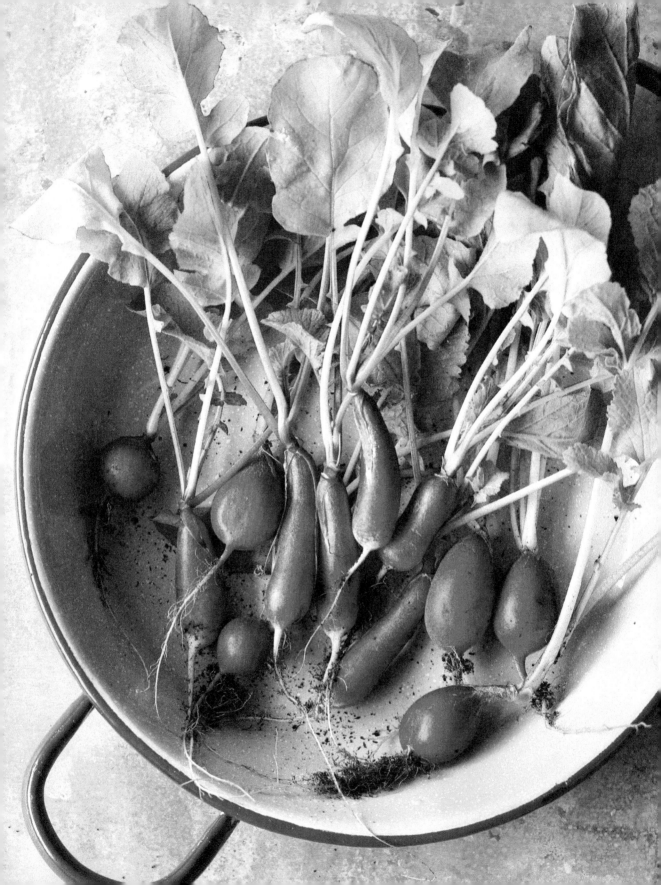

CONVERSION TABLES

VOLUME EQUIVALENTS (LIQUID)

US STANDARD	US STANDARD (OUNCES)	METRIC (APPROXIMATE)
2 tablespoons	1 fl. oz.	30 mL
¼ cup	2 fl. oz.	60 mL
½ cup	4 fl. oz.	120 mL
1 cup	8 fl. oz.	240 mL
1½ cups	12 fl. oz.	355 mL
2 cups or 1 pint	16 fl. oz.	475 mL
4 cups or 1 quart	32 fl. oz.	1 L
1 gallon	128 fl. oz.	4 L

OVEN TEMPERATURES

FAHRENHEIT	CELSIUS (APPROXIMATE)
250°F	120°C
300°F	150°C
325°F	165°C
350°F	180°C
375°F	190°C
400°F	200°C
425°F	220°C
450°F	230°C

VOLUME EQUIVALENTS (DRY)

US STANDARD	METRIC (APPROXIMATE)
⅛ teaspoon	0.5 mL
¼ teaspoon	1 mL
½ teaspoon	2 mL
¾ teaspoon	4 mL
1 teaspoon	5 mL
1 tablespoon	15 mL
¼ cup	59 mL
⅓ cup	79 mL
½ cup	118 mL
⅔ cup	156 mL
¾ cup	177 mL
1 cup	235 mL
2 cups or 1 pint	475 mL
3 cups	700 mL
4 cups or 1 quart	1 L

WEIGHT EQUIVALENTS

US STANDARD	METRIC (APPROXIMATE)
½ ounce	15 g
1 ounce	30 g
2 ounces	60 g
4 ounces	115 g
8 ounces	225 g
12 ounces	340 g
16 ounces or 1 pound	455 g

THE DIRTY DOZEN *and* THE CLEAN FIFTEEN

A nonprofit environmental watchdog organization called Environmental Working Group (EWG) looks at data supplied by the US Department of Agriculture (USDA) and the Food and Drug Administration (FDA) about pesticide residues. Each year it compiles a list of the best and worst pesticide loads found in commercial crops. You can use these lists to decide which fruits and vegetables to buy organic to minimize your exposure to pesticides and which produce is considered safe enough to buy conventionally. This does not mean they are pesticide-free, though, so wash these fruits and vegetables thoroughly.

These lists change every year, so make sure you look up the most recent one before you fill your shopping cart. You'll find the most recent lists, as well as a guide to pesticides in produce, at EWG.org/FoodNews.

DIRTY DOZEN

Apples	Nectarines	*In addition to the Dirty Dozen, the EWG added two types of produce contaminated with highly toxic organophosphate insecticides:*
Celery	Peaches	
Cherries	Spinach	
Cherry tomatoes	Strawberries	
Cucumbers	Sweet bell peppers	Kale/Collard greens
Grapes	Tomatoes	Hot peppers

CLEAN FIFTEEN

Asparagus	Eggplant	Onions
Avocados	Grapefruit	Papayas
Cabbage	Honeydew melon	Pineapples
Cantaloupe	Kiwis	Sweet corn
Cauliflower	Mangos	Sweet peas (frozen)

RESOURCES

APPS

FODMAPS

HealthyFood: FODMAP, Gluten, GMO Ingredient Scanner, by e-Med Tools

Low-FODMAP Diet 7-Day Plan—A Perfect Low-FODMAP Diet Food Plan with Grocery List, by Bhavini Patel

The Low-FODMAP Diet for IBS, by instamedic

The Monash University Low-FODMAP Diet, by Monash University

HEARTBURN AND GERD

Heartburn, GERD, and Acid Reflux Diary, by cellHigh

GLUTEN

Gluten-Free Fast Food Allergies Bundle, by awesomeappscenter

Gluten-Free Restaurant Items, by awesomeappscenter

Is That Gluten-Free? by Garden Bay Software

The Gluten-Free Scanner—Barcode Scanner, by Lluis Guiu

FOOD ALLERGIES

Bulletproof Food Detective by The Bulletproof Executive

mySymptoms Food & Symptom Tracker by SkyGazer Labs Ltd.

WEBSITES

FODMAPS

FODMAP Friendly Food Program: http://fodmapfriendly.com

IBS Diets FODMAP Food List: www.ibsdiets.org/fodmap-diet/fodmap-food-list

Monash University Low-FODMAP Diet: www.med.monash.edu/cecs/gastro/fodmap

ORGANIZATIONS

International Foundation for Functional Gastrointestinal Disorders (IFFGD): www.iffgd.org

Irritable Bowel Syndrome Self Help and Support Group: www.ibsgroup.org

The Center for Health and Healing: http://healingdigestivedisorders.org

The IBS Network: www.theibsnetwork.org

INSPIRATION

Byron Katie (inquiry into thoughts and beliefs): http://thework.com/en

The Center for Mindful Eating: http://thecenterformindfuleating.org/

BOOKS

Low-FODMAP 28-Day Plan: A Healthy Cookbook with Gut-Friendly Recipes for IBS Relief (Rockridge Press, 2014).

Reclaim Your Life from IBS: A Scientifically Proven Plan for Relief without Restrictive Diets, by Melissa G. Hunt, PhD (Sterling, 2016).

The Flexible FODMAP Cookbook: Customizable Low-FODMAP Meal Plans & Recipes for a Symptom-Free Life, by Karen Frazier (Rockridge Press, 2016).

REFERENCES

Allergy UK. "What Is Food Intolerance?" British Allergy Foundation. Last updated April 2016. Accessed February 13, 2017. www.allergyuk.org/food-intolerance /what-is-food-intolerance.

American Psychiatric Association. *Diagnostic and Statistical Manual of Mental Disorders (DSM-5)*. Arlington, VA: American Psychiatric Association, 2013. www.psychiatry.org.

Celiac Disease Foundation. "Irritable Bowel Syndrome, Gluten-Related Disorders, and the Low-FODMAP Diet." February 3, 2016. Accessed February 13, 2017. https://celiac.org/blog/2016/02/irritable-bowel-syndrome-gluten-related -disorders-and-the-low-fodmap-diet.

Food Allergy Research and Education (FARE). "Food Allergy Basics." Accessed February 13, 2017. www.foodallergy.org/about-food-allergies.

Food Allergy Research and Resource Program, University of Nebraska-Lincoln Institute of Agriculture and Natural Resources. "Prevalence of Food Allergies." Accessed February 13, 2017. http://farrp.unl.edu/resources/gi-fas/prevalence-of -food-allergies.

Hamilton Health Sciences. "Low Fermentable Carbohydrate Diet." August 5, 2015. Accessed February 13, 2017. www.hamiltonhealthsciences.ca/documents /PatientEducation/LowFermentableCarbDiet-trh.pdf.

Hunt, Melissa G., PhD. *Reclaim Your Life from IBS: A Scientifically Proven Plan for Relief without Restrictive Diets*. New York: Sterling, 2016.

International Foundation for Functional Gastrointestinal Disorders (IFFGD). "About IBS." Accessed February 13, 2017. www.aboutibs.org.

Ibid. "What Is IBS?" Accessed February 13, 2017. www.aboutibs.org/what-is-ibs.html.

Ibid. "What Causes IBS?" Accessed February 13, 2017. www.aboutibs.org /what-is-ibs-sidenav/what-causes-ibs.html.

Ibid. "Stress and IBS." Last updated June 15, 2016. Accessed February 13, 2017. www.aboutibs.org/what-is-ibs-sidenav/stress-and-ibs.html.

Isolauri, E., S. Rautava, and M. Kalliomäki. "Food Allergy in Irritable Bowel Syndrome: New Facts and Old Fallacies." *Gut* 53, no. 10 (October 2004): 1391–3. doi:10.1136/gut.2004.044990.

Magge, Suma, and Anthony Lembo. "Low-FODMAP Diet for Treatment of Irritable Bowel Syndrome." *Gastroenterology and Hepatology* 8, no. 11 (November 2012) 739–745.

Mayo Clinic Staff. "Irritable Bowel Syndrome Causes." Mayo Clinic. Accessed February 13, 2017. www.mayoclinic.org/diseases-conditions/irritable-bowel -syndrome/basics/causes/con-20024578.

Monash University, "Low FODMAP Diet for Irritable Bowel Syndrome." Accessed February 13, 2017. www.med.monash.edu/cecs/gastro/fodmap.

Myers, Amy, MD. "Do You Know What's Really Causing Your IBS?" November 27, 2015. Accessed February 13, 2017. www.amymyersmd.com/2015/11/whats -causing-your-ibs.

Nanayakkara, Wathsala S., Paula M. L. Skidmore, Leigh O'Brien, Tim J. Wilkinson, and Richard B. Gearry. "Efficacy of the Low-FODMAP Diet for Treating Irritable Bowel Syndrome: The Evidence to Date." *The Journal of Clinical and Experimental Gastroenterology* 9 (June 2016): 131–142. doi:https://doi.org/10.2147/CEG.S86798.

Robillard, Norm. "Could IBS Be an Autoimmune Condition?" Digestive Health Institute. February 19, 2014. Accessed February 13, 2017. https://digestivehealthinstitute .org/2014/02/19/ibs-autoimmune-condition.

"Syndrome." Dictionary.com. Dictionary.com, n.d. Web. 03 Apr. 2017.

Ruigómez, A., M. A. Wallander, S. Johansson, and L. A. García Rodríguez. "Irritable Bowel Syndrome and Gastroesophageal Reflux Disease in Primary Care: Is There a Link?" *Digestive Diseases and Sciences* 54, no. 5 (May 2009): 1079–1086. doi:10.1007 /s10620-008-0462-0.

The IBS Network. "Is It Food Intolerance?" Accessed February 13, 2017. www.theibsnetwork.org/diet/is-it-a-food-intolerance.

Vann, Madeline R., MPH. "GERD and IBS: What's the Connection?" Everyday Health. Last updated June 12, 2013. Accessed February 13, 2017. www.everyda yhealth.com/gerd/gerd-ibs-connection.aspx.

WebMD. "IBS Triggers and How to Avoid Them." Accessed February 2017. www.webmd.com/ibs/guide/ibs-triggers-prevention-strategies#1.

WebMD. "Irritable Bowel Syndrome (IBS)—Cause." Accessed February 13, 2017. www.webmd.com/ibs/tc/irritable-bowel-syndrome-ibs-cause.

RECIPE INDEX

INDEX

Ingredients
    low-FODMAP substitutions, 21–22
    pantry staples, 19–20
Inquiry process, 9
International Foundation for Functional
    Gastrointestinal Disorders (IFFGD), 2, 7
Intestinal tract, 2–3, 7
Intolerances, food, 4, 16
Irritable bowel syndrome (IBS)
    about, 2
    causes and triggers, 2–3
    dietary changes to reduce symptoms, 15–17
    factors that worsen, 3–4, 7
    and FODMAPS, 4–6
    high-FODMAP foods to avoid, 11
    low-FODMAP foods to enjoy, 12–13
    moderate-FODMAP foods to taste, 14
    stress and, 7–10

J

Jalapeño peppers, 98, 102–103
Journal of Clinical and Experimental
    Gastroenterology, 1

K

Kale, 51, 97
Katie, Byron, 9
Kitchen equipment, 17–18
Kiwis, 146

L

Lactose, 5–6
Lamb, 129
Leeks, 65, 150, 152
Lemons and lemon juice, 67, 96, 100, 104,
    105, 117, 135, 136, 157, 158, 159, 164
Lentils, 66, 86
Lettuce, 44, 46, 89
Limes and lime juice, 79, 95, 98,
    102–103, 114, 126, 154

Low-carb recipes, 26, 27, 34, 35, 39, 40, 44,
    45, 49, 50, 51, 52, 53, 55, 56, 64, 67, 78,
    80–81, 82, 91, 96, 97, 98, 99, 100, 101,
    102–103, 106, 107, 109, 112, 113, 117, 119,
    124, 125, 127, 128, 134, 136, 137, 138, 140,
    144, 145, 146, 150, 151, 152, 153, 154, 155,
    156, 157, 158, 159, 160, 161, 162, 163, 164
    about, 23

M

Macadamia nuts, 31, 159
Meats. *See also* Beef; Lamb; Pork
    FODMAPS food tables, 11–14
Melons, 30, 31, 134
Mindfulness meditation, 10
Monash University, 3, 6
Monash University Low-FODMAP
    Diet app, 6, 10
Monosaccharides, 5
Monterey Jack cheese, 72, 83
Mozzarella cheese, 46, 91
Myers, Amy, 3

N

Negative thoughts/feelings/reactions, 8–9
Nightshades, 16
Noodles, 62, 79. *See also* Pasta
Nuts and seeds. *See also specific*
    FODMAPS food tables, 11–14
    pantry staples, 20

O

Oats, 32, 84, 141
Oligosaccharides, 5–6
Olives, black, 44. 77, 164
Oranges and orange juice, 29, 47,
    53, 97, 106, 156, 161

V

W

Y

Z

ABOUT THE AUTHOR

KAREN FRAZIER is a freelance writer who has authored several cookbooks for people on special diets. Her previous books include *The Hashimoto's 4-Week Plan, The Acid Reflux Escape Plan, The Flexible FODMAP Cookbook,* and *The Hashimoto's Cookbook and Action Plan,* among others. Karen has learned to control her celiac disease, autoimmune conditions, and multiple food sensitivities through lifestyle and dietary changes. Karen lives in western Washington near Seattle with her husband and four dogs.

CPSIA information can be obtained
at www.ICGtesting.com
Printed in the USA
BVOW10s1439151017
497620BV00004B/4/P